# AGE *Healthier*
# *Live* HAPPIER

For more information, please write:
CelebrityPress®
520 N. Orlando Ave, #2
Winter Park, FL 32789
or call 1.877.261.4930

Visit us online at: www.CelebrityPressPublishing.com

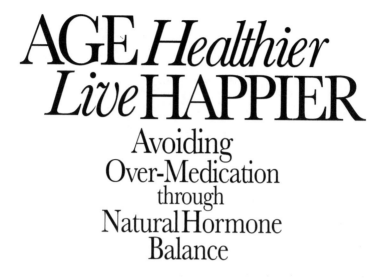

# AGE *Healthier* *Live* HAPPIER

## Avoiding Over-Medication through Natural Hormone Balance

*By*
## Gary Donovitz M.D.

*Foreword By*
## Dr. Neal Rouzier

CELEBRITY PRESS®
Winter Park, Florida

# CONTENTS

# CHAPTER 8

# CHAPTER 9

# ACKNOWLEDGMENTS

To my wife, Marci, who has been with me for eighteen years now. Through many ups and downs of my life including the stress that accompanies pioneering projects like this, she has been the stabilizing rock, including the disorder that accompanies pioneering projects like this. She is the mother of my son Chase, my personal organizer, chief critic, and my best friend. Chase is six years old but very interested in this book, asking all the questions I cannot answer yet.

To my daughter, Mandy, who has been such a great protégé in my quest to change healthcare. She has a heart of gold and is the most caring nurse, soon to be nurse practitioner I know. She has been my cheerleader, literally, for years and the bright light in my soul forever.

Thank you to Thomas Hauck and Angie Swenson with Celebrity Branding Agency who have helped me tell my stories and made them coherent for all to understand. Thomas has the keen ability to transfer ideas from my head and transcribe them onto paper. Thanks to Joe Kenrick for prompting me to write this book and leading me to Celebrity Branding Agency.

I am so pleased with the beautiful and creative cover design from my friend Christian Sly, you did an amazing job with the photography and capturing the spirit of my book!

There are others who were part of the journey and helped me see things through the eyes of women and the struggles of patients I may have missed. Thank you!

Finally, I would like to thank my patients. Over thirty years they have trusted me to help them. They have taught me what works and what does not. They have shared their stories, challenged me to keep them aging healthier, and rewarded me by sending all their friends and family to me.

# FOREWORD

Writing a book to educate and entertain both physicians and patients is a difficult and formidable task as they both think and want differently. However, I am both a physician as well as a patient and therefore understand the thought processes and desires of both. And therefore I write this Foreword from the perspective of a physician as well as a happy, healthy, content and optimized patient. Dr. Donovitz dreamed of writing such a book that addresses the needs of both physicians and patients alike, and he hits a home run with *Age Healthier, Live Happier.*

Dr. Donovitz has been teaching, preaching, and researching hormones for over 20 years and who therefore could possibly be better suited than he to enlighten us on HRT. Dr. Donovitz summarizes for us all his research, teaching, experience and medical studies to educate us how to improve and maintain our health and well-being. Although Dr. Donovitz has experience with all types of HRT as a board certified OB/GYN physician, after 20 years of research and experience he has discovered that HRT administration via pellet therapy works the best and therefore pellet therapy is his *forte* for administering bioidentical hormones (BHRT). Dr. Donovitz's experience with treating over twelve thousand patients with pellets, and training nearly one thousand practitioners at his monthly state-of- the-art training courses leads to him being the world's expert on pellets. His passion for teaching, impeccable knowledge, tremendous expertise with pellet administration and training makes Dr.

Donovitz a leader in the field of hormone replacement. Who better to write a book for patients and physicians to introduce them to all the health and wellness benefits of BHRT.

Thank you Dr. Donovitz for finally writing a book that reviews and explains the controversies and complexities of hormones for us all to understand. Medical studies and literature support are that which we physicians require in order to believe and embrace a concept or therapy. Patients require case examples, anecdotes, patient testimonials, and translation into simple language to thoroughly understand the importance of BHRT. *Age Healthier, Live Happier* accomplishes both. More importantly, patients and physicians will come to understand that patients no longer want to go to physicians only to be treated for a disease or illness, rather patients now demand that physicians partner with them to prevent disease and improve how we feel and function. Dr. Donovitz utilizes the medical literature to show how BHRT prevents disease and illness and at the same time make patients feel and function at their optimum.

Optimization of hormones is a strange and foreign concept for physicians to grasp as we are only taught to treat disease and illness. Optimizing our hormones with BHRT is not part of that realm. Patients are interested in preventing disease and illness but we are more importantly interested in feeling better, a concept that we physicians fail to comprehend as that is not what we are taught. *Age Healthier, Live Happier* helps educate us and bridges the gap from what we don't know but should know about our medical literature. And once we physicians become our own patients and finally appreciate how well we can feel on hormones, then we physicians finally understand how tremendous we can make our patients feel once we feel well ourselves. Dr. Donovitz is the expert at making a patient feel their best as can be seen from the patient testimonials. He is also the world's expert in training us physicians how to successfully treat our patients to feel their best. Also, in spite of the medical literature being confusing and contradictory, Dr. Donovitz explains the complexities of the studies, the faults, the misinterpretations, and how to correctly interpret these studies so we can make sense from all the HRT chaos. He reviews what happens to us when we lose our hormones, the benefits of replacing those hormones to optimum, and the harm of synthetic hormones.

To age, deteriorate, lose strength, energy, and sexual function and feel lousy is commonly treated by physicians with a pat on the back and an antidepressant – which is not what patients want or need. Yet most of us physicians first learn of HRT optimization from some patient that proclaims how fabulous they look and feel after being treated by Dr. Donovitz. This euphoria seen in our patients peaks our interest enough to go through the BioTE pellet training courses. And once that we physicians experience making our patients feel fantastic, then physicians like myself can't wait to tell the world how Dr. Donovitz has changed our lives, the lives of our patients, and our medical practices. The number one reason that doctors state they go into medicine in the first place is to help people. That is what makes the practice of medicine so special. There is no other therapy, treatment, drug, or otherwise that even comes close to that seen with BHRT. More importantly, as Dr. Donovitz so eloquently reviews and discusses in his training courses for physicians, there is no better preventive medicine then BHRT to protect against the illnesses of aging.

Dr. Donovitz also provides us with his background and path he followed, his trials and tribulations, and his success in becoming one of the world's leaders in teaching and guiding us to be superb in our treatment of patients. Dr. Donovitz is a master at orchestrating individualized treatment programs where he teaches us all the protocols for safe and effective administration of pellet therapy. In this book, Dr. D covers the background of BHRT pellet therapy and the technical data that we physicians demand that demonstrates the safety and efficacy of pellet therapy. Although many of us BHRT physicians are taught and practice BHRT, there are downsides with standard BHRT in achieving and maintaining efficacious serum levels as well as with compliance. Dr. D explains the option that eliminates all the other drawbacks of the standard therapies.

Hopefully someday you will have the pleasant opportunity to hear Dr. D lecture on BHRT. He is humorous, succinct, informative, entertaining, very knowledgeable, and so very passionate about BHRT. He uses our science and medical literature to guide us as to what we should be doing from a physician's perspective, what works, what doesn't work, and what is required based on EBM for optimal health and wellness. From a patient's perspective he explores the misleading conclusions and misinterpretations of the medical media that so confuses us practitioners as well as us patients. Most importantly he takes issue with medical academies that recommend only synthetic HRT in low doses for short-term use, which increases morbidity and mortality in every one of us due to hormone deprivation. Dr. D emphasizes that not all we hear or are taught is true as he utilizes the medical science to make sense out of the hormone phobia. He also makes physicians feel guilty when we ignore or reject all the medical literature support for superior outcomes in health when we optimize our hormones.

There are multiple methods for taking or administering BHRT. Dr. D introduces and supports medically that which is the safest and most efficacious method of monitoring and optimizing BHRT to maintain constant and therapeutic levels – pellet therapy. It is evidenced-based medicine with over 80 years of studies demonstrating superior outcomes and results. Dr. D teaches the most sought after and popular pellet training course. He is truly the doctor's doctor as he has trained over a thousand physicians with his method – which is well-researched and proven effective over the last 20 years. This is not the first book on BHRT, but it is the first to explore and explain pellet therapy.

For physicians it is not a matter of if you will ever do pellet therapy, but when. For patients, it is only a matter of time before your physician offers it to you as the preferred method for administration of BHRT. This book is for physicians as well as patients who want to understand the concept of helping our bodies operate maximally and how to maintain optimal hormone levels. This book is for all of us that need resources to support and validate the benefit of BHRT and pellet therapy. Dr. D assures anyone that doubts BHRT and pellet therapy with outcome studies, data, and references to support his therapy.

Thank you, Dr. D, for being the pioneer that pieces all this information together in a format for us all to enjoy and understand. And thank you for using your passion to bring BHRT to the forefront for both patients and physicians to provide us with better health care and quality of life as we age. Dr. Donovitz was also a pioneer in developing other beneficial procedures for women's health as with endometrial ablation, pelvic sling surgery, and robotic surgery. Now he is the most respected researcher and instructor for pellet therapy – which you will see in this book – as he takes us down a path to better health and wellness that your own family doctor may never understand.

Dr. Neil Rouzier
– *International Lecturer on*
  *Bio-Identical Hormone Therapy*
– *Director, The Preventative Medicine*
  *Clinics of The Desert*

# CHAPTER 1

# LIVING LONGER, FEELING SICKER

You stand before the mirror. It could be in the morning before you go to work, or in the evening as you get ready to go to bed.

You look at yourself.

The hair is thinner, the waistline bigger. You lean closer to the glass. Have some new wrinkles appeared next to the corners of your eyes? And your teeth—maybe you should get them capped, you think. That would be a big improvement.

Sure, you're not as young as you used to be. Who is? Getting older is a fact of life that people have been dealing with as long as human beings have been capable of thinking about life and death.

People are living longer than ever before, you say to yourself. Life is good—I don't want to complain!

But deep down inside, you don't feel right. You don't feel good.

It's more than just a new wrinkle or a bit of flab where you don't want it. You feel as though something is fundamentally wrong with the direction of your life.

The problem is not necessarily your job or your family. It's your *health* that's got you worried.

You open your medicine cabinet. There they are, lined up like soldiers going into battle: the little plastic bottles of the prescription drugs you take every day. Drugs that your doctor has prescribed for you. You read the labels of these best-selling medications:

- Levothyroxine, a hypothyroid medication
- Lipitor, which lowers cholesterol
- Esomeprazole, a proton-pump inhibitor to help with gastro-esophageal reflux Lexapro, an anti-depressant
- Metformin, to combat high blood sugar from adult onset diabetes mellitus
- Ambien, to help you sleep

Sometimes it's hard to keep track of them all.

You like your doctor. He or she listens patiently as you describe how you feel—tired, anxious and irritable, achy, and not sleeping well. He notes that you could stand to lose a few pounds and get more exercise. He may even have scheduled a battery of tests for you:

- EKG and other heart screening tests
- Bone scans for osteoporosis
- An MRI for low back pain
- Diagnostic tests for suspected allergies
- CT scans and other imaging procedures for headaches

None of these tests have revealed anything terribly wrong. Everything is within normal limits for a person of your age and gender.

Before you leave the examining room, your kindly doctor takes out his prescription pad, scribbles something, and hands it to you. "This will clear up your symptoms," he says. "I'd like to see you again in six weeks for a follow-up."

Yet all of these tests and prescription medications never seem to do any good. Oh sure, when your doctor prescribed a statin to reduce the level of cholesterol in your blood, after a few weeks your "numbers" got better. Your LDL (the "bad" cholesterol) went down, and HDL (the "good" cholesterol) went up a little bit. Your doctor warned you about the drug's potential side effects, which can include intestinal problems, liver damage, muscle inflammation, memory loss, mental confusion, high blood sugar, and Type 2 diabetes. But it seemed to be worth it, because you know from seeing the ads on television that having high cholesterol is a terrible thing that needs to be corrected at any price.

Sometimes you feel as though you're overmedicated and over-tested, and nothing seems to get better. Is it your imagination? Probably not. If you feel a deep sense of malaise, you are not alone. There are millions of Americans who don't feel well and don't know why. They're endlessly tested and medicated, but still they are sick.

## A TSUNAMI OF DRUGS

A 2013 Mayo Clinic study found that nearly seventy percent of Americans are on at least one prescription drug, and more than half take two. Published online in the journal *Mayo Clinic Proceedings*, the study revealed that one of five patients are on five or more prescription medications. Researchers found antibiotics, antidepressants, and painkilling opioids are the most commonly prescribed. Except high blood pressure drugs, which are more often used after the age of thirty, drugs are prescribed to both men and women across all age groups. Overall, women and older adults receive more prescriptions. Women receive more prescriptions than men across several drug groups, especially antidepressants. Nearly one in four women ages fifty to sixty-four are on an antidepressant. Among young and middle-aged adults, antidepressants and opioids are most common. Older adults get cardiovascular drugs, anti-diabetic drugs and drugs to make them sleep.

Is this progress? You think back to the old days. You remember hearing about your great-grandfather who, at the age of sixty, contracted pneumonia. He took to his bed. A week later he was dead. Just like that. Boom. Here one day, gone the next. That's how it was back then. People tended to get sick and then die much more quickly. To bring perspective to all of you, a century ago menopause and its male counterpart andropause marked the end of the lifespan. Now women and men will live more than thirty years longer.

## QUALITY OF LIFE

We live longer, but is our quality of life maintained? No, longevity has won out, but QOL has been continually discounted. Over the past century, breathtaking medical advances have been made. Introduced in the 1950s, polio vaccine has nearly wiped out this crippling disease. Ditto for smallpox. Doctors now perform amazing transplants and other operations that in great-grandpa's day were the stuff of science fiction.

Consequently we have more years, but what kind of years? Are they more time to really live, or more time to feel lousy?

For all of its advances, medicine seems to not work for us. Death still claims us. In the United States, the leading causes of death are heart disease, cancer, chronic lower respiratory diseases, and stroke (cerebrovascular diseases). Many of us die from accidents, and then the next most common causes of death are Alzheimer's disease, diabetes, influenza and pneumonia, and a trio known as nephritis, nephrotic syndrome, and nephrosis, or kidney disease. We are becoming increasingly overweight; over one-third of Americans are obese, and another one-third are overweight. These rates have more than doubled since the nineteen-seventies.

According to the World Health Organization, in 2013 the United States ranked thirty-fifth among nearly two hundred nations in overall life expectancy. Thirty-fifth! With an average of 79.8 years of individual life, we lag behind Japan (84.6), Italy (83.1), France (82.3), Israel (82.1), Germany (81)—practically every industrialized nation. We are even bested by Slovenia (80). Are you proud of that?

As you stare into the mirror and run your fingers across the plastic pill bottles in your medicine cabinet, you feel as though your doctor and the pharmaceutical companies whose cinema-quality ads flood the airwaves are only treating your symptoms. They are not *healing* you. Deep down inside, you're as sick as you've ever been.

Why? Why are we so sick? Here are some of the reasons.

## THE PERSISTENCE OF CARDIOVASCULAR DISEASE

Each year, cardiovascular disease is America's leading health problem, and the leading cause of death. According to the American Heart Association, approximately eighty-four million Americans suffer from some form of cardiovascular disease, causing about 2,200 deaths a day. That's one death every forty seconds. An estimated fifteen million U.S. adults have coronary heart disease, seventy-eight million have high blood pressure, and an estimated twenty million have diabetes. Cardiovascular disease is the cause of more deaths than cancer, chronic lower respiratory diseases, and accidents combined. It's the number one killer of both women and men.

The direct and indirect costs of cardiovascular disease and stroke are about $315 billion, and this figure is increasing every year.

What causes cardiovascular disease? While the term can refer to many different types of heart or blood vessel problems, it's often used to mean damage caused to your heart or blood vessels by *arteriosclerosis*, which is the term for when the blood vessels that carry oxygen and nutrients from your heart to the rest of your body become thick and stiff, restricting blood flow to your organs and tissues.

*Atherosclerosis* is a specific type of arteriosclerosis that refers to the buildup of fats, cholesterol and other substances in and on your artery walls (plaques), which can restrict blood flow.

25

Atherosclerosis is the most common cause of cardiovascular disease, and it's often caused by an unhealthy diet, lack of exercise, being overweight or obese, and smoking. All of these are major risk factors for developing atherosclerosis and, in turn, cardiovascular disease.

## OBESITY

Even as many parts of the developing world experience persistent food insecurity, its opposite, obesity, is becoming a worldwide epidemic. In the United States, the prevalence of *overweight* (body mass index [BMI] 25 to 29.9) and *obesity* (BMI 30 and above) is over sixty percent. Obesity can also be more simply defined as having a waist circumference of forty inches (102 cm) or more for men and thirty-five inches (89 cm) or more for women, although waist circumference cutoff points can vary by race. Obesity is also on the rise in most other industrialized countries.

But what does this mean? Is it unhealthy to be fat? What are the consequences?

It depends who you ask. Founded in 1969, the National Association to Advance Fat Acceptance (NAAFA) says it is a "non-profit, all volunteer, civil rights organization dedicated to protecting the rights and improving the quality of life for fat people. NAAFA works to eliminate discrimination based on body size and provide fat people with the tools for self-empowerment through advocacy, public education, and support." NAAFA asserts that "our thin-obsessed society firmly believes that fat people are at fault for their size and it is politically correct to stigmatize and ridicule them."

Be that as it may, the actual and measurable health risks of being overweight or obese—for whatever reason—are well documented. Excess weight and obesity are linked to *metabolic syndrome*, which is a cluster of conditions including increased blood pressure, a high blood sugar level, and abnormal cholesterol levels that, when occurring together, increase your risk of heart disease, stroke, and diabetes.

A central feature of metabolic syndrome is insulin resistance, which results in hyperglycemia and hyperinsulinemia, and can eventually lead to the development of diabetes.

Having just one of these conditions doesn't mean you have metabolic syndrome. However, any of these conditions increase your risk of serious disease. If more than one of these conditions occur in combination, your risk is even greater.

According to the Third National Health and Nutrition Examination Survey (NHANES III), in 2014 the prevalence of metabolic syndrome in the United States was twenty-three percent in persons aged twenty years or older, and over forty percent in those who were aged sixty and older.

If you have metabolic syndrome or any of the components of metabolic syndrome, significant lifestyle changes can delay or even prevent the development of serious health problems.

## DIABETES

Hot on the heels of the increase in obesity has come a global increase in diabetes.

Diabetes begins with insulin, a hormone that is produced in the pancreas. Insulin facilitates the transfer of glucose (blood sugar) from the bloodstream into our body's cells. Our cells need glucose as fuel. Without glucose in our cells, they would not be able to function. Without the appropriate levels of insulin, glucose stays in your bloodstream, raising your blood sugar level. High blood sugar, or hyperglycemia, can lead to the signs and symptoms of diabetes.

In *insulin resistance*, muscle, fat, and liver cells do not respond properly to insulin and thus cannot easily absorb glucose from the bloodstream. As a result, the body needs higher levels of insulin to help glucose enter cells. The pancreas tries to keep up with this increased demand for insulin by producing more. Over time, insulin resistance can lead to Type 2 diabetes and prediabetes because the pancreas fails to keep up with the body's increased need for insulin. Without enough insulin, excess glucose builds up in the bloodstream, leading to diabetes, prediabetes, and other serious health disorders. (Prediabetes is a condition where blood glucose levels are higher than normal but not high enough to be called diabetes.)

There is a clear but as yet undefined causal relationship between obesity and insulin resistance. Although the exact causes of insulin resistance are not completely understood, scientists think the major contributors to insulin resistance are excess weight, hormone imbalance, and physical inactivity. The *location* of your body fat seems to be important. Individuals with greater degrees of central adiposity (the accumulation of fat in the lower torso around the abdominal area) develop this syndrome more frequently than do those with a peripheral body fat distribution.

These circumstances lead to diabetes, which is a group of metabolic diseases in which the individual has high blood glucose (blood sugar), either because the body's cells do not respond properly to insulin, or because insulin production is inadequate, or a combination of both. Patients with high blood sugar will typically experience polyuria (frequent urination), they will become increasingly thirsty (polydipsia) and hungry (polyphagia). Why does this matter to you? For two reasons:

*The first reason is that diabetes is a serious disease.* According to the World Health Organization (WHO), the consequences of diabetes include:

- Increased risk of heart disease and stroke. Fifty percent of people with diabetes die of cardiovascular disease (primarily heart disease and stroke).

- Combined with reduced blood flow, neuropathy (nerve damage) in the feet increases the chance of foot ulcers, infection and eventual need for limb amputation.

- Diabetic retinopathy is an important cause of blindness,

and occurs as a result of long-term accumulated damage to the small blood vessels in the retina.

- Diabetes is among the leading causes of kidney failure.
- The overall risk of dying among people with diabetes is at least double the risk of their peers without diabetes.

*The second reason is that diabetes is becoming epidemic.* The number of Americans diagnosed with diabetes rose from 1.5 million in 1958 to 18.8 million in 2010, an increase of alarming proportions. Roughly 79 million adults aged twenty and older have prediabetes. Diabetes is the seventh leading cause of death in the United States, and among people with diabetes, cardiovascular disease is the leading cause of death. It is estimated that one in three Americans living today will eventually develop diabetes, and that the number of cases will increase in this country by 165% by 2050.

Not surprisingly, diabetes has become big business. There are an estimated 370 million people in the world with diabetes. More children are developing the disease and more people are dying from diabetes, and so more and more people are seeking treatment. Standard & Poor's has estimated the annual market will increase from $35 billion in 2014 to $58 billion by 2018. As *The Motley Fool*, an investing website, recently said, "Drugs in this space have the potential to reach blockbuster status, and companies are consequently clamoring for market share. In particular, GLP-1 (glucagon-like peptide-1) agonists mimic an endogenous incretin hormone that spurs the body to produce more of its own insulin; these agents hold the distinct advantage of being either once-a-day or weekly dosing. The field is becoming more crowded, with Novo Nordisk's blockbuster Victoza, AstraZeneca's Byetta and Bydureon, and Sanofi's once-daily Lyxumia."

If you listen carefully, you can almost hear countless pens scratching out more prescriptions on the pads of doctors from sea to shining sea.

## IODINE DEFICIENCIES

Iodine? Isn't that the stuff they put in salt? The orange liquid your mom put on your cut when you were a little kid?

Yes, and for good health you need it in your diet. Essential to life, iodine is especially crucial for brain development in children, making its deficiency the number one cause of preventable mental retardation worldwide. It also plays an important role in healthy function of your thyroid gland. This is why the most visible symptom of iodine deficiency is *goiter*—the painful enlargement of the thyroid gland that manifests as an unsightly swelling around the neck and larynx.

The problem is that in nature, iodine is a relatively rare element. While it's found in abundance in the ocean, its presence in soil is very low in many places around the world, including the United States.

Not long ago, this was a problem that was considered solved, at least in industrialized nations. In the 1920s, salt iodization was implemented to counteract the effects of iodine deficiency. Iodine was added first to flour, then to salt, and the problem was considered solved. While goiter was relatively common a few generations ago, nowadays most Americans have never seen it.

Less than a century later, there is an epidemic of iodine deficiency in this country that affects every man, woman and child, and especially vegetarians. Over the last thirty years our iodine intake has declined by fifty percent, while the ingestion of toxic competing halogens such as bromine, fluorine, chlorine, and perchlorate has dramatically increased in food, water, medicines, and the environment.

In the 1960s, iodine was added as an anti-caking agent to bakery products, but because of misplaced fears of iodine toxicity ("iodophobia"), in the 1980s it was replaced with bromine, the gas used to fumigate houses for termites. Bromide is also widely present in soil and crop fumigants as well many foods and drugs.

Perchlorate is a key ingredient in rocket fuel. It continually makes its way up the food chain through ground and drinking water, into feed and edible plants, animal products, milk, and breast milk, and can now be found in virtually all humans tested. Perchlorate blocks the thyroid gland's ability to absorb and utilize dietary iodine, an effect that is of concern when iodine intake drops off.

Research suggests these halides compete with iodide for absorption and uptake in the body. This means they function as *goitrogens*, or substances that suppress thyroid function by interfering with iodine uptake and accumulation.

In addition, because of medical advice to cut our salt intake, we're consuming less table salt, which is generally iodized. We're still eating vast quantities of salt in processed foods, but this salt does not contain iodine. By cutting our salt intake we are also cutting our iodine intake, which is why research has revealed that mean urinary iodine levels (a measure of iodine sufficiency) have dropped by more than half over a twenty-year period.

It is this iodine deficiency that has led to the increased risk of breast cancer, prostate cancer, Hashimoto's thyroiditis, and so many other contemporary health issues. You can take steps to avoid iodine deficiency by consuming foods rich in iodine, including sea vegetables (kelp, dulce, nori), yogurt, cow's milk, eggs, strawberries, mozzarella cheese, iodine-containing multivitamins, iodized table salt, saltwater fish, shellfish, soy milk, and soy sauce. The reality is we need much more iodine than our recommended daily allowance told to you by the federal government.

## OVERMEDICATED SENIORS

As we live longer, we're taking more drugs. This is such a common occurrence that it even has a name: Polypharmia. That's the term used to describe older patients who take more drugs than they actually need.

Many Americans with an aging parent have experienced this scenario. Mom or Dad isn't feeling well. They may even seem to be "not themselves." Out of curiosity, you go to their medicine cabinet. Inside you find shelves of pill bottles, all of them prescription. Some may be from multiple doctors. Who can take so many pills and not get sicker?

The problem is so widespread that physicians are now consulting the *Beers Criteria for Potentially Inappropriate Medication Use in Older Adults*, commonly called the *Beers List*, which is a guideline for healthcare professionals' to help improve the safety of prescribing medications for older adults. Originally published in the *Archives of Internal Medicine* in 1991 and since updated, it emphasizes de-prescribing medications which are unnecessary to healthcare.

There were more than fifty-five million prescriptions for opioid painkillers given to people over sixty-five years of age in 2013 alone. It is reprehensible that over 100,000 emergency room visits last year were for misuse of medications by our seniors.

## THE END OF HORMONE REPLACEMENT THERAPY

Sometimes, a safe and effective treatment is unfairly maligned by poorly designed studies, leading to its needless discontinuance by people who are benefitting from it.

Pioneered in the 1940s, hormone replacement therapy (HRT) became more widely used in the 1960s, leading to advances in the management of menopause. HRT was prescribed to menopausal women for the relief of symptoms including hot flashes, night sweats, sleep disturbances, psychological and genito-urinary problems, and for the prevention of osteoporosis.

In 2002, a national study asserted that the combination estrogen-progestin regimen used by millions of middle-aged and older women—an estimated six million of them in the United States alone—did more harm than good.

Funded by a National Institutes of Health program called the Women's Health Initiative (W.H.I.), the study was begun in 1993 with over 16,000 participants. Originally scheduled to continue well into 2005, the trial was stopped in 2002 because, after an average 5.2 years of participant follow-up, it was claimed that increased cases of invasive breast cancer were found among those taking the hormone regimen than in women taking a placebo.

Then in 2003, the so-called Million Women Study (MWS) provoked headlines when it said hormone replacement therapy (HRT) led to a rise in breast-cancer incidence. Based on questionnaires returned by more than a million post-menopausal women in Britain, its estimate caused a wave of anxiety and much confusion among regulators and doctors and among women using HRT.

But an assessment published in 2012 in the *Journal of Family Planning and Reproductive Health* revealed the design of the MWS study had so many problems that a safe conclusion could not be drawn. "HRT may or may not increase the risk of breast cancer, but the MWS did not establish that it does," the paper said bluntly.

Today, many so-called "experts" have conceded that for the majority of women who use HRT for the short-term treatment of symptoms of the menopause, the benefits of treatment are considered to outweigh the risks. Unfortunately, these "experts" continue to overlook the numerous published studies on the *long-term* benefits of hormone replacement therapy.

Men and women are not being told that long-term hormone replacement therapy can decrease their risk for heart disease, diabetes, Alzheimer's disease, breast cancer, and osteoporosis.

In 2013, the *American Journal of Public Health* reported that since the flawed data of the Women's Health Initiative was published in 2002 and restated in 2012 by the same physicians who knowingly deceived the public, tens of thousands of women have died because they stopped their hormones.

So yes we are living longer, too bad the quality of our life is disintegrating. If we want to co-pilot our health on the go forward, we must see who are our friends and who is our foe. Is it possible to change medicine from a business to a profession of healthcare restoring the health and vitality for all of us?

## CHAPTER 2

# BIG PHARMA AND THE BUSINESS OF MEDICINE

If you're over the age of forty, you probably remember the television show *Marcus Welby, MD*. From 1969 to 1976, Robert Young came into our living rooms as a family practitioner with a kindly bedside manner. Dr. Welby was the perfect family doctor: personable, empathetic, and possessing vast medical knowledge. His intuitive way of treating patients was contrasted against the more strait-laced methods of his young colleague, Dr. Steven Kiley, played by James Brolin.

In the very first episode, Dr. Welby has the opportunity to give a speech to a group of young interns. It is anticipated that most of them will choose not to become general practitioners but specialists instead.

"General practice is performed standing up, sitting down, outdoors, indoors, wherever there's illness," said Dr. Welby. "And that means everywhere. Because, gentlemen, we don't treat fingers or skin or bones or skulls or lungs. We treat people. Entire human people.

"I hope some of you will go into general practice. For if you don't, where will a patient turn who doesn't know that he has an orthopedic problem? Or a neurological problem? Or a psychiatric problem? Or a nutritional problem? He only knows that, in lay terms, he feels lousy."

There is nostalgia for the family doctor, who now treats patients less often than he or she acts as a gatekeeper to the vast and growing universe of specialists. When you feel lousy, and you dutifully follow the rules of your HMO by visiting your primary care physician, your doctor is less likely to treat you than give you the coveted referral to a specialist—someone you cannot approach on your own, at least not if you expect your HMO to foot the bill.

There's a good reason for the explosion of specialists. In the days of Marcus Welby, most patients suffered from acute, often infectious conditions that required prompt attention. That has changed. Today the majority of patients have complex quality of life (QOL) conditions such as coronary artery disease, diabetes, obesity, lung cancer, strokes, and chronic degenerative diseases. In the past, it made some sense to organize health care into subspecialties that would treat acute, easily-diagnosed conditions. But patient health has changed. By the time a patient needs a cardiologist, a surgeon, an oncologist, or an endocrinologist, his or her condition has become a complex set of QOL factors that have much deeper roots than the highly-focused "fix" provided by the specialist.

As a result, money is spent on focused fixes that fail to address the underlying problems. Then more money is spent on more fixes. And people still feel lousy.

Our patchwork health care system of competing private enterprises is difficult to reform or even control. Primary care physicians know that there's too little time to care adequately for patients, too much bureaucratic paperwork, and no access to the big money pulled down by specialists.

In America, medicine has gone from being the practice and art of healing to an industry. Our healthcare system accounts for more than $2.5 trillion in annual expenditures, which is nearly twenty percent of the US gross domestic product (GDP). By 2020, healthcare spending is projected to exceed $4.5 trillion.

## BIG PHARMA

A big chunk of this vast marketplace is occupied by the pharmaceuticals industry. According to the World Health Organization (WHO), the global pharmaceuticals market is worth $300 billion a year, a figure expected to rise to $400 billion within three years. The ten largest drug companies—commonly known as Big Pharma—control over one-third of this market, and several post sales of more than $10 billion a year with profit margins of thirty percent.

If you were a visitor from Mars, you might think that the gargantuan size of the global pharmaceuticals industry would provide hope and comfort to those who are sick. After all, for every ailment under the sun, there's a pill. There are even pills for diseases that you may not know you have. But the vast flow of money into the coffers of Big Pharma is not wholly directed towards helping people become healthy. Much of it, in fact, is turned around and spent on efforts to get consumers to buy *more* pills, either over the counter or by convincing their doctors to write prescriptions.

Dr. Arnold Relman, *professor emeritus* of medicine and social medicine at Harvard School of Medicine, and past editor of *The New England Journal of Medicine*, reported that Big Pharma spends one-third of all sales revenue on marketing their products—roughly twice what they spend on research and development.

As a result of this drive to maintain sales, there is now, in the words of WHO, "an inherent conflict of interest between the legitimate business goals of manufacturers and the social, medical and economic needs of providers and the public to select and use drugs in the most rational way."

## MARKETING TO CONSUMERS

If you watch television, you see it for yourself every day. Big Pharma now pitches drugs directly to consumers, who then go to their doctors and say, "I've heard about this drug. I think it will help me."

How did the advertising floodgates open? We can pinpoint the two causes.

**Cause #1:** Prior to 1997, the rules of the US Food and Drug Administration (FDA) said, "Advertisements promoting the medical use of prescription drugs must contain a 'brief summary' of all important information about the advertised drug, including its side effects, contraindications, and effectiveness. In addition, advertisements broadcast over radio, TV or through telephone communications systems must include a 'major statement' prominently disclosing all of the major risks associated with the drug."

Requiring a "major statement" made TV ads for prescription drugs impractical. Television was not a cost-effective way to market drugs.

In August of 1997, the FDA quietly relaxed the rule. The change allowed the drug companies to "include information about any major risks, as well as instructions for how consumers can easily obtain more detailed information about the drug's approved uses and risks." Now an advertiser could simply provide a mechanism to ensure that consumers could easily obtain full product labeling. In other words, it became enough to quickly list some of the negative side effects along with a toll-free phone number or web address, and to advise the viewer to speak with their physician.

**Cause #2:** At the beginning of this century, both government regulators and physicians' groups became increasingly concerned about the cozy relationship between Big Pharma and individual physicians and hospitals. Big Pharma had developed a culture of aggressive marketing of drugs to doctors at all levels, in the hopes that the physicians would write prescriptions. No expense was spared: endless free samples, trinkets, office supplies, conventions in resort areas, dinners and clubs. The pressure on doctors was relentless.

As the American College of Physicians reported in 2008, hospitals began to tighten rules on gifts, meals, and "education" from Big Pharma. Conflict of interest policies were revised, primarily at academic medical centers, and affected everything from free food and office supplies to funding for continuing medical education. The *ACP Hospitalist* reported that "pharma-funded lunches have become a thing of the past at many academic medical centers, including Yale, Stanford and Boston University, and one hospital has gone so far as to send every item that carries a drug logo to Africa.... Many of the recent efforts to build barriers between the pharmaceutical industry and hospital staffs can be traced back to a 2006 policy proposal for academic medical centers that was published in the *Journal of the American Medical Association.*"

Kenneth Irons, MD, chief of community clinics for SMDC Health System in Duluth, Minn., an organization that purged all its pharma trinkets, said, "We wanted to make sure, for our patients, that we eliminated the perception that we were significantly under the influence of the pharmaceutical industry. We wanted to make sure that the information that we were using in our prescription decisions was as unbiased as possible."

There has been action on the federal level. First introduced in 2007 by U.S. Senators Charles Grassley and Herb Kohl, the Physician Payment Sunshine Act requires that all manufacturers of drugs, devices, and biological and medical supplies covered by federal health care programs collect and track all financial relationships with physicians and teaching hospitals. The goal of the law is to enhance patient safety by increasing the transparency of financial relationships between health care providers and pharmaceutical manufacturers. The act did not pass in Congress, but eventually became part of the Patient Protection and Affordable Care Act, commonly called the Affordable Care Act (ACA) or Obamacare, which was signed into law by President Barack Obama on March 23, 2010.

Faced with increasingly tougher restrictions on direct access to physicians, and the loosening of requirements for television ads, Big Pharma pivoted away from selling to physicians and went directly after consumers. That's why every time you turn on your TV, you're subjected to a barrage of ads for drugs to treat diseases that you never knew you had.

The ads are produced and presented with the quality approaching mini-feature films. They present a reliable scenario: the drug-taking consumer doing daily activities that he or she is not able to do as well without the drug.

The sales pitches use two angles of attack:

The first is fear: the drug can *prevent* something bad from happening to you, such as a stroke or heart attack. You may *feel* healthy, but you are *not* healthy. The actor always says, "I never saw it coming! Suddenly I had a heart attack! I thought I was healthy!" You may feel fine, but deep inside your body, your arteries are clogged. You're a heart attack waiting to happen, so you'd better take preventive action. Every part of your body—your bones, your eyes, your muscles, your joints—is subject to failure, especially as you grow older. If you're smart, you'll take the pill or the one-monthly injection. Why would you gamble with your health?

The second angle of attack is *curative:* The pill can cure an identifiable disease that threatens you. The message is that it's a short step from your state of unhealthiness to health. Are you short of breath? See how this person—your peer—can now breathe easily. Can't get an erection? See how this guy—who looks much too young to have such a problem—confidently snuggles his beautiful wife. Do you suffer with persistent heartburn because you overeat? Not to worry; a prescription antacid pill will allow you to continue to stuff yourself with five thousand calories a day.

In their TV advertisements, drug companies must provide a general disclaimer of possible negative side effects. This is no problem for the producers of drug ads. The soothing tones of the voiceover actress deliver the possible side effects— "shortness of breath, nervousness, loss of appetite, sleeplessness, heart attack, and death"—while the visuals show the happy patient engaged in swimming or golfing or hiking. The effect is powerful and intoxicating. Those side effects aren't happening to the actor; why be afraid they will happen to you?

## SOPHISTICATED BRAND MANAGEMENT

The public rhetoric of Big Pharma would be comical if it were not creepy. The slogans used by top pharmaceutical companies say one thing, but in the end they follow the money.

### Pfizer

Founded by cousins Charles Pfizer and Charles Erhart in New York City in 1849 as a manufacturer of fine chemicals, Pfizer, Inc. is a multinational pharmaceutical corporation and the second-largest health care company (after Johnson & Johnson), with 2013 revenues of $51.6 billion.

Pfizer's products include many that you've seen advertised on television: the blockbuster Lipitor (*atorvastatin*), used to lower LDL blood cholesterol; Lyrica (*pregabalin* for neuropathic pain/fibromyalgia); Diflucan (*fluconazole*), an oral antifungal medication; Zithromax (*azithromycin*), an antibiotic; Viagra (*sildenafil*, for erectile dysfunction); and Celebrex/Celebra (*celecoxib*), an anti-inflammatory drug.

Pfizer loves to say that it's "Working for a Healthier World" and "Life Is Our Life's Work." The documented examples of Pfizer's hypocrisy would fill ten books; if you want to get a sense of what people say about Pfizer, just Google "Pfizer hypocrisy" and you'll be richly rewarded.

Here's just one example:
In 2006, Peter Rost, M.D., former vice president for Pfizer, published *The Whistleblower: Confessions of a Healthcare Hitman*. It was the first exposé written by a senior executive of one of the world's largest pharmaceutical companies. *The*

*Whistleblower* is a vivid unmasking of the illegal, even criminal business practices the author witnessed at his corporation, as well as his crusade to legalize the re-importation of drugs.

Here's what one commentator on Amazon posted about the book and about Pfizer:

"As a Pfizer employee, I am extremely upset by the facts laid out in Dr. Rost's book *The Whistleblower: Confessions of a Healthcare Hitman*. I had previously drank the 'Pfizer blue Kool-Aid.' An example: Pfizer has a number of 'values' and 'leader behaviors' printed on expensive, colorful posters and on cardboard mobiles which hang throughout the hallways of its skyscrapers and campus buildings. To think these values and leader behaviors are just for the little people—the rank and file workers—and that top Pfizer executives and management who strive to be promoted to the executive ranks are above ethical behavior will forever change how I view Pfizer. Pfizer's corporate tag line is 'Life Is Our Life's Work.' After reading Dr. Rost's book, they ought to scratch out the word 'life' and add the word 'hypocrisy' in there somewhere. If Dr. Rost's thrilling new book is true, I'm thoroughly disgusted by Pfizer's behavior towards honest employees."

In its aggressive manipulation of public opinion, Pfizer is hardly alone.

## Merck

In 2005, Merck & Co., based in New Jersey and with revenues of $27 billion, launched a new TV ad campaign costing $20 million in which the company proclaimed the slogan, "Merck—Where Patients Come First." As John Mack on his *Pharma Marketing Blog* said, "The veracity of this slogan might be on a par with other infamous slogans such as 'War is Peace' or 'Work Makes You Free.' " A Congressional committee exposed damning evidence that Merck had a specific program to train its sales reps on techniques for avoiding cardiovascular questions from doctors while presenting them with alternative data.

Merck is perhaps most well known for the Vioxx debacle. When Merck pulled the pain medication off the market in 2004, many admired the company's courage to do the "right thing" by putting people's lives before profits. A few days later it was revealed that Merck may have known about Vioxx's cardiovascular side effect problems for years, concealed the evidence, and blocked action by the FDA.

In November 2004, *The New York Times* reported that four years earlier, in May 2000, the company's top research and marketing executives met to consider whether to study the disturbing possibility that Vioxx, a hugely profitable painkiller, might pose a heart risk. Two months earlier, results from a clinical trial conducted for other reasons had suggested such a possibility. But the executives rejected pursuing a study focused on the cardiovascular risks of Vioxx. Merck's marketers feared it could send the wrong signal about the company's confidence in Vioxx, which already faced fierce competition from a rival drug, Celebrex.

"At present, there is no compelling marketing need for such a study," said a slide prepared for the meeting. "Data would not be available during the critical period. The implied message is not favorable."

On Sept. 30, 2004, after a second study confirmed the drug caused severe cardiovascular problems, Merck was forced to initiate a worldwide recall of Vioxx. However, by this time, up to twenty-five million Americans had taken Vioxx, with millions more having taken the drug worldwide.

Drugwatch.com reported that within weeks of the Vioxx recall, injured patients across the nation were seeking justice in court. With an abundance of cases, a federal multidistrict litigation (MDL) was established in Louisiana with nearly 50,000 claimants. Other claimants filed private lawsuits in state courts nationwide.

The company's shareholders threatened to sue as well, saying they lost billions because Merck had deceitfully marketed Vioxx. To settle consumer claims, Merck set up a $4.85 billion settlement fund and paid nearly 35,000 complaints. Financial settlements made with injured patients allowed for compensation in accord with injuries. Of the 20,591 heart-attack claims, which included 2,878 deaths, payments ranged from $18,000 to $1.79 million. For the 12,447 valid stroke claims, including 590 related deaths, settlements ranged from $5,000 to $820,000.

## AstraZeneca

In January 2007 *Medical Media Marketing* reported that AstraZeneca (based in Sweden, with revenues of $32.8 billion) was rolling out a spiffy new ad slogan: "Healthcare For People, Imagine That." AstraZeneca's commercials focused on what it was doing to help treat individual patients. The company said that it was "putting the personal touch back in healthcare."

## Bristol-Myers Squibb

"Together We Can Prevail" is the slogan launched by Bristol Myers Squibb (revenues $18 billion) in 2008. One of BMS's commercials features a cancer survivor, Sharon Blynn, who founded "Bald is Beautiful," a cancer advocacy organization. BMS used the commercials to talk about its commitment to fighting "serious diseases." Lance Armstrong also participated in the campaign.

But according to DrugWatch.com, during the first decade of this century the company faced legal trouble over deceptive advertising campaigns and FDA violations. BMS has also had to deal with litigation related to two of its successful diabetes products, Byetta and Bydureon.

In 2001, BMS reportedly persuaded wholesale customers to buy $2 billion more of drugs than they wanted so the company could meet its sales goal that year. This accounting trick, known as "channel stuffing," resulted in a decrease in revenue the following year and triggered investigations by the SEC and Justice Department. The company agreed to pay a total of $839 million in restitution.

In 2007, BMS agreed to pay more than $515 million to settle a broad array of cases involving its drug pricing and marketing. In addition to overcharging the government for drugs, Bristol was accused of setting inflated prices for a wide array of drugs and promoting off-label use of the antipsychotic, Abilify.

## THE PHARMACEUTICAL RESEARCH AND MANUFACTURERS OF AMERICA

Founded in 1958 and based in Washington, D.C., the Pharmaceutical Research and Manufacturers of America (PhRMA) represents the country's leading biopharmaceutical researchers and biotechnology companies. The organization's website says, "Our members are committed to finding tomorrow's cures and treatments for some of the most serious diseases such as cancer, Alzheimer's disease, cystic fibrosis and Parkinson's. New medicines are an integral part of the healthcare system, providing doctors and their patients with safe and effective treatment options, extending and improving quality of life."

**PhRMA's mission is this:**
To conduct effective advocacy for public policies that encourage discovery of important new medicines for patients by pharmaceutical and biotechnology research companies. To accomplish this mission, PhRMA is dedicated to achieving these goals in Washington, the states and the world:

- Broad patient access to safe and effective medicines through a free market, without price controls.
- Strong intellectual property incentives.
- Transparent, effective regulation and a free flow of information to patients.

In January 2007, PhRMA began airing commercials featuring talk show host Montel Williams. In the advertisements, Williams touted the Partnership for Prescription Assistance (PPA), a patient assistance program the pharmaceutical industry launched in April 2005. In addition to airing spots for PPA, a number of drug companies, including Pfizer, aired commercials focusing on their scientific mission and quest to help patients.

It was a rocky partnership. *The Wall Street Journal* reported that Williams showed up in Savannah, Georgia to promote PPA. By the time he left town, the talk show host had threatened to "blow up" some local reporters, according to the *Savannah Morning News*.

The threat was apparently triggered by the following question, posed by a high school intern working as a reporter: "Do you think pharmaceutical companies would be discouraged from research and development if their profits were restricted?"

Williams, who has multiple sclerosis, abruptly ended the interview.

Later in the day, the same reporter went to a local hotel on an unrelated story. Williams, who was at the hotel for a separate event, believed he had been followed there. Williams apparently approached him and said, "Don't look at me like that. Do you know who I am? I'm a big star, and I can look you up, find where you live, and blow you up." Not exactly the image PhRMA wanted to project. PhRMA didn't fire Williams; as of this writing he's still the PPA spokesperson.

The mission and goals of PhRMA are not science-based free enterprise but rather slight-of-hand, and their rhetoric is full of empty arguments. The industry group claims high prices are necessary incentive to discover innovative drugs. Where are those innovative drugs? What they give doctors and patients are "me too" drugs backed by mind-crushing marketing campaigns.

PhRMA claims that whatever the cost for prescription drugs may be, we're getting our money's worth. In reality, we're falling fast on the world stage in how we rank in performance in healthcare and how we rank in quality life expectancy. Since profits exceed expenditures on research and development, lowering the cost of pharmaceuticals, especially the "me too" drugs, would not affect R & D budgets.

PhRMA and its Big Pharma members use their wealth to wheel-and-deal through American political lobbying, obtaining favoritism, control and big profits. In 2013, they spent $226 million lobbying Congress using more than 1,400 lobbyists. According to the website: opensecrets.org, this leads all private sector companies.

If pharmaceutical companies are focused on healthcare and prevention, then it's difficult to see why we have the problems described in Dr. John Abramson's book, *Overdosed America: The Broken Promise of American Medicine*. They cover:

- The relative performance of US Healthcare, measured in terms of improvement in overall healthcare, has declined since 1960.

- Overall life expectancy in the US ranks 29th amongst all nations.

- Americans pay 70% more for prescription drugs than Canadians and Western Europeans.

- According to the FDA, of the 569 new drugs approved in the US between 1995 and 2000, only 13% actually contain a new active ingredient that offers a significant improvement in already-available drugs and therapies.

- Less than 25% of the "new" drugs had any significant improvement over products that were already on the market.

An area of great concern is the cozy relationship between the U.S. Food and Drug Administration (FDA) and the companies of PhRMA. The 1992 Prescription Drug User Fee (PRUFR) mandated that drug companies pay a fee to speed up FDA approval of drugs. According to the Institute of Medicine, that fee now accounts for 50% of the FDA's budget. *Therefore, the FDA is dependent on the industry it is supposed to regulate.*

There's a huge conflict of interest as pharmaceutical companies direct the medical treatment, do the clinical research and/or fund it, and do the physician education. Conflicts of interest translates into biases that affect physician prescribing. The victim is the patient.

Big Pharma holds itself out as a major platform of discovery. That's a myth; the reality is that public funding through the National Institute of Health (NIH) is responsible for many of our medical advances. The bottom line is that the global companies of the pharmaceutical industry are not creating cures. They are creating customers.

CHAPTER 3

# HORMONES—THE FOUNDATION TO GOOD HEALTH

The human body is a complicated machine. You know the basics—our bodies are built with a skeleton, muscles, organs, a brain, and many systems. The building blocks of all of these components are the individual cells. By the most the current estimate published in the *Annals of Human Biology*, an adult human is composed of roughly 37.2 trillion cells. These cells work more or less harmoniously to maintain human life and let you do all the stuff that you do every day. (Your 37.2 trillion cells also provide a happy home for the roughly 100 trillion microorganisms that live in your gut—but that's a subject for another book.) Your cells come in a wide variety of shapes and sizes, which is one reason why it's difficult for scientists to count them. In case you're interested, the largest and smallest cells in the human body are both part of the reproductive system. The largest cell in the human body is the female ovum or egg, which is roughly one millimeter across and barely visible to the naked eye. The smallest is the male equivalent of the female gamete, commonly known as the sperm cell, or spermatozoon, which is only sixty micrometers in length. (A micrometer is 1/1000 of a millimeter.) Sperm cells are not visible to the naked eye, and you need a microscope to examine them.

It's one of the miracles of life that our 37.2 trillion human cells plus our 100 trillion microbial tenants manage to work together to achieve an average life span for someone living in the United States of 78.74 years. The good news is our lifespan is increasing, which is why this book is so important so you know how to "age healthier" and avoid harmful synthetic drugs!

The task of managing and directing the countless activities of our cells—moving, thinking, communicating, eating, reproducing—falls to a number of systems in our bodies. The most obvious, of course, is the brain, which, as the body's chief executive, controls a large proportion of what we do every day.

But there are other systems that work behind the scenes to regulate and manage our bodies' many complex biochemical processes. These systems do not require conscious thought; they just happen naturally as the result of our organic programming. You do not consciously digest your food or make your heart beat; these involuntary actions are controlled by unseen instructions. For example, when you cut your finger, the bloodstream rushes white blood cells to the damaged area to help fight off infection. It's a service that your body provides without conscious direction.

## HORMONES AND HEALTH

One of the important regulatory systems embedded in your body's apparatus is your portfolio of hormones. These are chemicals that your body has synthesized. They act as messengers, designed to interact with specific target cells and organs and provoke a change or result. Hormones are found in all multi-cellular organisms and their role is to provide an internal communication system between cells located in distant parts of the body. Hormones are secreted directly into the bloodstream, which carries them to organs and tissues of the body to exert their functions. Some of these functions include:

- Cognitive function and mood.
- Development and growth of the body.
- Digestion and metabolism of food materials.

- Maintenance of body temperature and thirst.
- Reproductive growth and health.

Hormones are secreted from specialized endocrine glands in the body. The glands are ductless, which means that many hormones are secreted directly into the blood stream rather than by way of ducts. Some of the major endocrine glands in the body include:

- Pituitary gland
- Pineal gland
- Thymus
- Thyroid
- Adrenal glands
- Pancreas
- Testes
- Ovaries

For example, the pituitary gland is located in the brain. This gland reaches its maximum size in middle age and then gradually becomes smaller. The front (anterior) portion of the pituitary gland produces hormones that affect the thyroid gland (TSH), adrenal cortex, ovaries, testes, and breasts.

The hypothalamus is also located in the brain. It produces hormones that control the other structures in the endocrine system. While the amount of these regulating hormones stays about the same, as we age the response by the endocrine organs can change.

The thyroid gland is located in the neck. It produces hormones that help control metabolism. Beginning at around age twenty, metabolism begins to slow down.

The parathyroid glands are four small glands located around the thyroid. Parathyroid hormone affects calcium and phosphate levels, which affect the strength of the bones. Parathyroid hormone levels rise with age, which may contribute to osteoporosis.

The pancreas produces insulin, which facilitates the transfer of sugar (glucose) from the blood to the cells, where it can be used for energy.

The adrenal glands are located just above the kidneys. The adrenal cortex, the surface layer, produces the hormones aldosterone and cortisol. Aldosterone regulates fluid and electrolyte balance. Aldosterone release decreases with age, which can contribute to light-headedness and a drop in blood pressure with sudden position changes (orthostatic hypotension). Cortisol is the "stress response" hormone.

The ovaries and testes produce the sex hormones that control secondary sex characteristics, such as breasts and facial hair. They also perform hundreds of other functions, which we will cover in detail later.

Some hormones, such as insulin and growth hormones, are fully active when released into the bloodstream. Others must be activated in specific cells through a series of activation steps that are highly regulated.

While all of the body's cells are exposed to all of the hormones circulating in the bloodstream, not all cells react to them. Hormones affect specific target tissues by binding to receptor proteins to elicit a specified action in the cellular target. Conversely, cells respond to a hormone when they express a specific receptor for that hormone.

## CHANGES IN OUR HORMONES

Because it takes very low levels of hormones to bring about major changes in the body, hormones are secreted in microscopic amounts. Either a very slight excess of hormone secretion or the slightest deficiency can lead to disease states.

The levels of various hormones fluctuate on both a short-term basis—hour-by-hour, day-by-day—as well as on a long-term basis over many years and even over our lifetimes. Some of the most significant long-term changes occur as we age from maturity into what used to be called our "golden years." Change happens at both ends of the hormonal system: Over time, the amount of hormones produced may change, while some target tissues may become less sensitive to their controlling hormone. Blood levels of some hormones increase, some decrease, and some are unchanged. Hormones are also broken down (metabolized) more slowly.

Many of the organs that produce hormones are, in turn, controlled by other hormones. Aging changes this process. For example, an endocrine tissue may produce less of its hormone than it did at a younger age, or it may produce the same amount at a slower rate. In addition, the receptors for these hormones change as we age. They are often affected by the toxins we put in our bodies.

The state of our health is directly related to the state of our hormones. While individual health varies greatly, there are typical ages at which hormones begin to decline. By age thirty, both men and women enter what's called somatopause. This is when the human growth hormone (HGH) begins its decline. Falling about fourteen percent per decade after the age of thirty, by the age of eighty, production of HGH has been reduced to five percent of what it was at the age of twenty.

Typical signs and symptoms of decreasing HGH in your body could include low energy, reduced muscle strength, weight gain or loss, mood swings, sagging skin, poor memory, greying hair, fluctuation in blood pressure, slow wound healing, diminished libido, and sleep difficulties.

Women enter perimenopause. The term means "around menopause," and refers to the time period during which a woman's body begins its transition toward permanent infertility and sex hormone deprivation (menopause). Women start perimenopause at different ages—in their thirties or forties and sometimes sooner. The perimenopause usually commences ten to fifteen years before menopause. During perimenopause, the level of estrogen rises and falls unevenly. A woman's menstrual cycles may lengthen or shorten, and she may begin having menstrual cycles in which her ovaries don't release an egg. Additionally, a women's testosterone level begins to fall. She may develop symptoms of anxiety, irritability, depression, weight gain, muscle aches, fatigue, reduced sex drive, insomnia, poor memory focus and concentration, and night sweats (not to be confused with the hot flashes of menopause). She may also experience symptoms resembling menopause, such as hot flashes, sleep problems and vaginal dryness. DHEA levels (dehydroepiandrosterone) begin to decrease. This occurs mostly because the adrenal gland is capable of producing testosterone, and in trying to replenish the testosterone levels it becomes overworked. Hence the term "adrenal fatigue." The good news is that the adrenal gland usually recovers after testosterone is replenished.

After age forty, many women enter menopause. This is the age when progesterone, and estrogen begin to decrease. Progesterone begins to fall in the late perimenopause and continues its decline as a women enters menopause. It's defined as having experienced twelve consecutive months without a period. However, it can be diagnosed much earlier, so there's often no need for a woman to suffer for an entire year.

Effects may include aches and pains in the joints, chronic fatigue, depression, sleep disturbances and anxiety. A woman begins losing bone mass and her cholesterol begins increasing. The decreasing amount of progesterone in the body can also be attributed to weight gain (in the form of fat and cellulite around the hips and thigh area), low libido, water retention, and indirectly cause hypertension.

Thyropause is a "season" within the "seasons" of perimenopause, menopause, andropause. The thyroid function begins to decline. This can occur at any age, and often begins in the twenties.

After age thirty-five, men may begin to experience andropause (the male version of menopause). Men, like women, go through a decline in hormones, namely testosterone and to a lesser extent DHEA. Libido and sexual performance may decrease, sleep and mood is affected, muscles and strength decrease, fatigue, weight gain, and a disturbance of the immune system function may occur. The body's ability to cope with sugar declines, and the insulin resistance or diabetes becomes more prevalent. The typical "middle-age spread" is due to the fact that the hormones no longer protect the body from the negative effects of the peaks and valleys in the sugar levels.

## FOCUS ON THE SEASONS OF OUR LIVES

These broad shifts in hormonal production and their effects have often been called "the seasons of our lives," not unlike spring, summer, fall, and winter. There are three fascinating seasons in our lives that are too often overlooked by the medical establishment: perimenopause and menopause in women, and andropause in men. Why is this? Perhaps it's because one hundred year ago, no one cared about these life cycle seasons. People most often died soon after reaching them. They were simply considered to be part of "old age" and a precursor of death. But today, we are living longer, and most of us will spend fully one-half of our lives either enjoying these years or dreading them.

As we age from the summer of our lives into fall and winter, how can we retain the good health and vitality of youth? How can we maintain the intricate functions of our bodies and avoid the onset of disease as we age?

As we've seen in the previous chapters, Big Pharma would have us consume increasing quantities of patented drugs, produced in laboratories and sold on TV, to combat the outward symptoms of the diseases of age: brittle bones, clogged arteries, sleeplessness, low libido, and weight gain. The specialists who staff our hospitals would treat us by fixing this broken part or that one, and sending a hefty bill to our HMO, who would pass the cost onto us, our employers, or the taxpayers.

And yet we still feel sick! Is it any wonder why we still feel unhealthy? Such measures do not treat the underlying changes that are obvious to any first-year medical student. We know that our hormonal levels change as we age; is it not a matter of common sense to first investigate our hormones to determine if these changes are a cause of disease?

To begin our investigation, let's begin with perimenopause, menopause, and andropause. Let's see how we can regain our lives and make these best seasons of our lives, full of vitality, great personal relationships, and better productivity at work.

For women, the three most important hormones that need to be considered in optimizing an individual's hormones providing longevity with outstanding quality of life and disease prevention are estrogen, testosterone and thyroid. For men, there are two, testosterone and thyroid.

### Estrogen
Estrogen is an amazing hormone. It has over four hundred functions in a woman's body. It protects the skin and keeps you looking young. It protects the nerves in the brain, reduces the risk of Alzheimer's disease, and has been shown to reduce the risk of heart disease. Unbeknownst to many, it is necessary to shed that unwanted "belly fat." Estrogen is also very important in properly remodeling your bones and avoiding osteoporosis.

### Testosterone
Testosterone is one of the most important hormones in both men and women (yes, women produce a lot of testosterone every day). Women start losing their testosterone production in their twenties, and men start losing theirs in their thirties. In males, low testosterone known as androgen deficiency in the adult male (ADAM) causes a host of problems: Increased risk for Alzheimer's disease, heart disease, osteoporosis (men get osteoporosis too!), prostate cancer, diabetes, and muscle loss. Women with low testosterone have similar issues: Increased risk for Alzheimer's disease, heart disease, osteoporosis and fractures, diabetes and metabolic syndrome, and possible increased risk for breast cancer.

Testosterone deficiency often results in many common complaints including loss of energy, loss of mental clarity, loss of muscle mass, weight gain (especially around the mid-section), difficulty losing weight even while exercising and eating appropriately, decreased exercise tolerance, anxiety, irritability, depression, bone loss, decreased sex drive in women, and loss of erectile ability in males. Optimal levels of testosterone not only allow patients to get in shape more quickly, but stay in shape with much less effort.

### Thyroid

The thyroid gland is located in the front lower part of your neck. Hormones released by the gland travel through your bloodstream and affect many parts of your body, including your heart, brain, muscles, and skin.

The thyroid controls how your body's cells use energy from food (also called your metabolism). Your metabolism affects many things including your heartbeat, your body's temperature, and how well you burn calories. If you don't have enough thyroid hormone, your metabolism slows down. That means your body makes less energy and you become sluggish, gain weight, and are less inclined to exercise.

Hypothyroidism, also called underactive thyroid disease, is a common disorder whereby the thyroid gland does not make enough thyroid hormone

As many as forty percent of Americans are hypothyroid. That's nearly fifty-two million people. What kinds of symptoms would you have if your thyroid levels were low? They might include fatigue, lethargy, sleepiness, depression, cold intolerance, dry skin, weight gain, joint pain, constipation, and high cholesterol. These symptoms may resemble those experienced with low testosterone.

### Progesterone

For women there is a "bonus hormone." It's not one that everyone recognizes as important and not one everyone thinks about. It's called progesterone. Not just any progesterone will do; it must be micronized progesterone. Unlike synthetic forms you would find in birth control pills and many forms of synthetic HRT used for menopause, natural micronized progesterone is a form of the hormone progesterone derived from plants, and which matches human progesterone. It's called "micronized" to describe how it's made using oil to encourage absorption through the digestive tract when taking capsules by mouth.

Many women feel micronized progesterone is more calming, helps them sleep, and complements their estrogen therapy very well, especially when compared to the side effects of synthetic progestins like Provera (*medroxyprogesterone acetate*). Natural micronized progesterone has beneficial effects on the heart including reducing atherosclerosis and cholesterol levels, reducing the risk of uterine cancer, reducing the risk of breast cancer, and improving cognitive function. One of its few side effects is somnolence, which can be a good thing because it helps you sleep at night.

Synthetic progesterone, like that used in the Women's Health Initiative, has adverse effects on your HDL cholesterol (the good one), the heart, and the brain. In addition, the synthetics increase swelling, bloating, anxiety, irritability, headaches, food cravings, depression, and muscle aches.

The bottom line is that if your doctor is not familiar with the benefits of micronized natural progesterone and tries to put you on synthetic progesterone, you owe it to yourself to politely but firmly decline.

## THE BENEFITS OF HORMONE OPTIMIZATION

Now that we know about the importance of hormones and how they can help people of both genders, let's look at individual parts of our bodies where the most benefits can be derived.

### Heart Disease

Heart disease remains the number one killer of both men and

women. One in seven premenopausal women die from heart disease. After menopause that number jumps to one in three. More than 200,000 women die each year from heart attacks, five times as many women as breast cancer. Coronary artery disease is also the number one killer of men.

Pharmaceutical companies would have all of us believe it's our cholesterol. But while statins have climbed the ladder to the number one selling medication in America, the number of heart disease related deaths is not decreasing. If you treated one hundred persons with statins, less than a handful of heart attacks would be prevented.

If we look at what happened after 1990, the picture becomes much clearer. Obesity is on the rise. One-third of the overall population is obese. Some ethnic groups have a higher rate; for example, thirty-six percent of Latin Americans have metabolic syndrome. The incidence of diabetes has doubled from 1990-1998 and continues to increase. As people live longer, more and more people are entering menopause and andropause; and as their hormones are depleted cholesterol goes up, blood pressure increases, and inflammation in their blood vessels goes up. You can see a storm brewing.

If we optimize the hormones that have been depleted in men and women, their weight decreases, their energy increases, and they feel like exercising again, which is a huge benefit to preventing heart disease. Hormone balance will restore blood flow to the coronary arteries, decrease plaque formation, and reduce inflammation in the blood vessels.

Bringing your testosterone in the optimum range reduces cholesterol and triglycerides, and increases HDL cholesterol. This means your lipids are getting back to normal without the harmful and less beneficial statins.

Some sources claim that testosterone causes an increase in heart attacks. It is just the opposite. There have been numerous studies showing that testosterone protects the heart. In 2013 the

*Journal of the American Medical Association* reported that men on testosterone had more heart attacks. A review of their own data revealed the opposite. There were fewer heart attacks in men taking testosterone, and nearly fifty percent fewer deaths. Most recently, in July 2014, in the *Annals of Phamacotherapy*, researchers from the University of Texas at Galveston performed a large study using testosterone in elderly men. Their results again showed a reduction of heart attacks in men using testosterone. A protective effect, if you will.

For women, not all progesterones are created equal. The micronized natural progesterone is protective to the heart by dilating blood vessels and improving the good HDL cholesterol. Unfortunately, many physicians are still giving patients synthetic progesterone, which has adverse effects on the heart.

Let's not forget the positive benefits of maintaining optimal thyroid balance. Hypothyroidism is a major contributor to heart disease. If your thyroid is optimized, you can prevent many heart attacks because thyroid fortifies your immune system and reduces inflammation, which reduces plaque formation and allows more oxygen rich blood to be pumped to your heart muscle.

There's no reason to take statins that decrease energy, cause muscle pain, decrease cognitive function, and increase the risk for diabetes. In many cases we can avoid using the anti-diabetic drugs that have numerous side effects and only put a band-aid on the problem. We can avoid fad diets and diet pills that are unhealthy for our thyroid and can increase our blood pressure and simply just don't work long term. In the future, we can say that by healthy life choices of exercising, stopping smoking and getting our hormones optimized, we actually have reduced the incidence of heart disease.

### The Brain

The number of cases of Alzheimer's disease is projected to triple by 2050. The cost to care for these patients will exceed one trillion dollars. Not to mention the tremendous burden they place on our loved ones who must also continue to care for them.

A very basic way of understanding Alzheimer's disease is that as nerves get stressed, they entangle. Once the nerve fibers get entangled, the brain lays down a substance called beta amyloid, and the degenerative process is now irreversible. Conventional drugs are minimally effective and expensive.

Parkinson's disease is also a neurodegenerative disease that affects millions of Americans. Rather than treating the symptoms, wouldn't you rather *protect* the nerves in your brain from neurodegenerative diseases like Alzheimer's and Parkinson's disease?

You can. When optimized, natural estrogen, natural testosterone, and natural progesterone protect the brain. Synthetics do not. When your hormones are depleted, the neurons of the brain suffer "oxidative stress" and the downward spiral starts. In addition, the nerves of the brain need energy. To make that energy, your body needs thyroid hormone. Not just any thyroid hormone but T3, which is the active thyroid hormone. How can you be sure your thyroid is optimal? Get your free T3 test, and make sure your doctor doesn't treat you with inactive synthetic thyroid hormones that may provide you with sub-optimal protection.

When in balance, the natural bio-identical hormones work as antioxidants. They decrease inflammation around the nerves, improve blood flow to your brain, and they decrease the production of that "bad" substance beta-amyloid. Prevention promotes healthier aging and happier life.

**The Bones**

Osteoporosis is a major problem. Twenty percent of women over the age of fifty have osteoporosis, and another forty percent have osteopenia. This thinning of the bones is a set-up for hip and vertebral fractures as we age. The National Osteoporosis Foundation have shown that twenty-four percent of people who suffer a hip fracture die within one year. Many of the others wind up living in assisted living centers and can no longer live alone.

Bone mineral density (BMD) can quickly and painlessly tell you whether you have osteopenia or osteoporosis. It is unfortunate that the American College of Obstetrics and Gynecology doesn't recommend testing until age sixty-five. Women start losing bone in perimenopause and could benefit from strengthening their bones in a very proactive fashion.

It's also unfortunate that the World Health Organization, funded by Big Pharma, defined osteopenia and osteoporosis BMD values such that millions of women would require treatment with expensive drugs that were unsafe and expensive. The bisphosphonates, as they would be called, cause abnormal remodeling, jawbone necrosis, heart arrhythmias, and severe nausea and vomiting. Did patients stay on them? Of course not! Did they change the absolute risk of fractures? Well, if you treated nearly one hundred women with bisphosphonates for four years, you would prevent one fracture. The cost would be more than $250,000!

If you look at data from the National Institute of Health—data not tainted by the pharmaceutical companies—you could prevent more than twice as many hip fractures using moderate exercise than using the high-priced, side-effect-riddled bisphosphonates.

Testosterone, estrogen, and thyroid are necessary for proper bone remodeling so that your risk for fractures is largely reduced. Vitamin D3 and Vitamin K2 are also important. Testosterone is the "bone builder." As will be discussed in the next chapter, hormone replacement therapy in women lacking testosterone will only decrease bone reabsorption, but not stimulate new bone growth. So for years women have been given the wrong hormones, in the wrong doses, and by the wrong route (orally), and they've still developed osteopenia and osteoporosis. Now you know why!

Thyroid helps maintain normal bone architecture by keeping the body from being too acidic. As we age and our bodies become too acidic, we leach calcium from our bones. That's why patients who take calcium alone don't build strong bones and never will. With proper hormone balance, bones remodel year after year, calcium is laid down appropriately thanks to Vitamins D3 and K2, and osteoporosis and osteopenia can be successfully ameliorated. And no harmful drugs are necessary.

## The Breasts

Breast cancer is the most common cancer in women. There are more than 400,000 deaths annually worldwide from breast cancer. Seventy-five percent of breast cancers occur in postmenopausal women. For years, women have been told after treatment for their breast cancer they should *not* take hormones.

After the data from the Women's Health Initiative, many women were led to believe that all hormones cause breast cancer. Fifty percent of primary care physicians quit prescribing hormone replacement therapy after that landmark 2002 article in the JAMA. Unfortunately for women, the data from the estrogen-only part of the study wasn't sensational enough to make the headlines. It showed that estrogen does *not* cause breast cancer. It was the synthetic progestin in the PremPro arm of the study where there was an increased risk.

In the *Journal of the National Cancer Institute* in 2001, hormone replacement therapy after a diagnosis of breast cancer was evaluated in relation to recurrence and mortality. Those women on hormone replacement therapy had fewer recurrences and fewer died.

It's time for myth to concede to reality. Natural hormones don't cause breast cancer. In fact, testosterone is breast protective and reduces the risk of breast cancer. Natural progesterone is also breast protective and reduces a women's risk of breast cancer.

## Type 2 Diabetes

Americans are in the midst of major health concern that has been growing like wildfire since 1990. Between 1990 and 1998 the number of people with Type 2 diabetes doubled. Over the past decade it has increased more than seventy-five percent. More than one million new cases of Type 2 diabetes are being recorded annually. Type 2 diabetes is the sixth leading cause of death in America. The health concerns are broad reaching, as this increases your risk for heart disease, kidney disease, vascular problems, and more.

If we look at the Nurses' Health Study published in the *New England Journal of Medicine* in 2001, being overweight, being sedentary, smoking, and having a poor diet were major contributing factors. In the *Journal of Sexual Medicine* in 2013, men with low testosterone were projected to add 1.1 million new cases of Type 2 diabetes.

The medical literature has done little to address prevention. Nearly every year there is a new drug to replace an old drug to treat Type 2 diabetes. The cost of these medications is high and the side effects severe.

As we age, both men and women lose testosterone. As this happens we begin to notice that we begin to gain weight around our midsection. This is because as we lose our testosterone, we develop insulin resistance. That means that it requires more insulin to metabolize our sugars and carbohydrates. The higher insulin levels lead to the increase in belly fat.

We can be proactive in our prevention of Type 2 diabetes by balancing and optimizing our testosterone. Then we can avoid the expensive and harmful drugs that conventional medicine and the pharmaceutical companies are marketing to us because we won't need them.

Clearly, to age healthier and live happier and more productive lives, we need to treat the disease of aging at its source by optimizing our hormones and making better lifestyle choices that include diet and exercise. What we don't need are pills, pills, and more pills fed to us by pharmaceutical marketing predators. Pills have a limited ability to improve our health and a much greater chance of creating further medical problems, leading to more medications, until we are all overmedicated and living unhappy lives.

The next chapter will explain how to optimize your hormones in the safest and most cost effective way possible.

CHAPTER 4

# BIO-IDENTICAL HORMONE REPLACEMENT FOR WOMEN —THE POSITIVE ALTERNATIVE

We've seen in previous chapters that even though we may be living longer, we aren't living longer and feeling better. I've shown the vast reach of the pharmaceutical companies, and how the tsunami of drugs that is flowing out of factories around the world and into our medicine cabinets is only adding to the problem, not solving it. Our manufactured society fills our minds with broken promises of treating symptoms, but never really solving the underlying problems. To add to the insanity, instead of addressing why these changes occur, advertising firms are hired by these companies to flood our televisions with countless commercials of middle-aged actors posing as happy life-fulfilled couples strolling on the beach hand-in-hand. It appears to be the perfect life.

It can be. Not with pills, pills, and more pills, but rather with a positive alternative. I have introduced you to your system of hormones, an amazing part of your body that keeps your 37.2 trillion cells working at top efficiency. It is a proven fact that as you age your hormone levels decline, making your body simply not work as well.

- What can you do to maintain and regain your health, vitality, and vigor?
- What can you do to enhance your relationship intimately?
- What can you do to actually age healthier and live happier?

65

Take drugs? No—that is not a good solution. Is it diet and exercise? Of course it is, but not entirely. We all know we must maintain proper nutrition by eating a variety of well-balanced food groups. And of course we have to exercise to keep our muscles toned and our hearts healthy. We can agree that diet and exercise play an important role in maintaining a healthy lifestyle. However, even the leanest diet and walks around the park cannot replenish what is already lost.

If a change in your hormone levels is the root cause of your feeling lousy, then it makes sense to attack the problem at its source.

*Your hormones. How do we do that?*

It's amazingly simple: a qualified physician provides you with bio-identical hormones to replace the amounts you've lost.

Why bio-identical? Bio-identical means that the hormone is an *exact molecular match* of your depleted human hormone. Your body cannot tell the difference. Before I get into the details, here's a case study that demonstrates the power of bio-identical hormones.

## CAROL AND ANNE

Carol and Anne are identical twins. Twenty-five years ago, when they were each thirty-five years old, they suffered from the same symptoms of depression, anxiety, irritability, mood swings, fatigue, weight gain, low libido, and sleeping difficulties. You might think that because they're twins, Carol and Anne would always do the same things. They'd dress alike, eat the same foods, and even seek the same medical treatment when they were sick.

That may be true to a certain extent, but when Carol and Anne felt chronically lousy, they didn't go to the same doctor. They each sought different treatments. Their choices provide a stark lesson in the problems with some of today's medical opinions and the treatments offered.

To address her health concerns, Carol chose to visit her primary care practitioner.

After a quick consultation, Carol's practitioner prescribed an anti-depressant to address two of her chief complaints, even though this class of drugs has been shown to decrease sex drive and cause weight gain.

Five years later—at age forty—Carol returned to her practitioner. Now addicted to anti-depressants, she had become increasingly overweight, and still had no sex drive and no energy. Concerned about the extra pounds, she asked for help and was prescribed a diet pill. She was worried about her increasing anxiety as well, so her doctor prescribed an anti-anxiety medicine and a sleeping pill for the sleep disturbances.

At age forty-five, Carol returned to her practitioner, still depressed and overweight. He noticed that her cholesterol was up. Rather than counseling her about lifestyle changes and examining her poly-pharmacy, he put her on a cholesterol-lowering drug called a statin, which has been shown to cause liver issues and muscle tissue breakdown. The fatigue and muscle pain discouraged her from pursuing an exercise routine, adding more pounds, which increased her depression.

Carol's exam at fifty years old fared no better. She complained of no menstrual cycle, hot flashes, and night sweats. She was put on an oral synthetic hormone pill, which has been shown in studies to increase risk of blood clots, heart attacks, strokes, and breast cancer. Her hot flashes were likely gone now, but she still had no sex drive or energy and was still overweight.

*Carol still felt horrible!*

At fifty-five, Carol told her practitioner she had quit taking oral hormones because she didn't like them. She was miserable, and on top of all her other symptoms she thought she was getting early Alzheimer's because she had memory problems. According to her bone density scan, she now had bone loss, and she was placed on a drug for bone building, which caused her severe nausea and chest pain. Her blood pressure was now high. She developed Type 2 diabetes and was placed on two additional medications.

By the time Carol turned sixty, because her doctor didn't understand how important hormone balance was to improving her mood, mental clarity, anxiety, bone building, heart health, diabetes prevention, weight control, breast cancer protection, and Alzheimer's disease prevention, she was tied to a lifelong ball and chain of medications that merely acted as a band-aid masking her symptoms rather than getting to the root cause of the problems. At age sixty, Carol is still tired, miserable, overweight, depressed, and irritable, can't think, has no sex drive, and is taking over ten different synthetic medications.

The story of her twin sister Anne is very different. Twenty-five years ago, feeling similar symptoms as her twin sister, Anne chose to seek out alternative answers. She felt her symptoms were hormonally related, so instead of following traditional treatments through her primary care physician, she sought the advice of a physician trained and qualified as a hormone balance expert.

After an in-depth consultation, her hormone expert agreed with her suspicions and narrowed down for her the options available to her for treating her hormone imbalances. She too was suffering from pre-menopausal symptoms of testosterone deficiency. Anne was very surprised to learn that women not only make testosterone in their ovaries, but it's a vital hormone for their overall physical and mental health and wellbeing.

After a simple blood test, it determined that Anne's suspicions were accurate. She was deficient in testosterone, low thyroid, and borderline levels of Vitamin D, all revealed by tests that her sister never received. Based on the research Anne had done on the subjects of hormone balance, hormone replacement therapy with bio-identical hormone pellets, and improvement in overall health, she opted to move forward with the therapy.

Two months after beginning hormone treatments, Anne returned to her hormone practitioner for a follow up. She could not believe how amazing she felt! The depression, anxiety, mood swings, and sleep issues were all gone, as well as the fatigue. And wow—what a libido!

Her husband prayed she never stopped this therapy. His wife was back! She was back in her workout routine and looked more like her old self.

At age forty-five, Anne was fit, lean, exercising, was on no extra medications, and her annual check-up was so amazing her primary practitioner (who also treated her twin sister) wanted to know what she was doing to stay in such great shape. She shared with him she was on a natural hormone balance therapy with bio-identical hormone pellet implants. Although he scoffed under his breath, he was intrigued by the differences between Anne and her twin sister.

At fifty-five, Anne's hot flashes and menstrual changes began. Not a problem for Anne! Her hormone balance practitioner simply added a bio-identical estrogen pellet to her testosterone therapy, along with some natural progesterone to balance her estrogen. Anne sailed through the perimenopause and menopause years with minimal, if any, setbacks. She avoided the pharmacy of prescription medications her sister was taking. Moreover, her baseline bone density scan was normal, her cholesterol levels were perfect, and her body mass index (BMI) and blood work were all within range. She showed no indication of diabetes and her blood pressure was normal.

While her primary care practitioner was still skeptical, he was beginning to see with his own eyes how beneficial this therapy had been.

At age sixty Anne feels great, looks great, has energy, mental clarity, sharp focus, and an amazing sex drive!

Anne was tired of being part of a healthcare system of drug

profiteering and disease management. To change this she had a paradigm shift in her mindset regarding her health, and she told herself, "I'm going to co-pilot my health. I'm not going to be overmedicated by the commercial interests of the pharmaceutical companies and physicians that are not on board with preventative healthcare."

Drug companies market drugs to consumers not because a market *exists*, but to *create* one. Reclaiming your life means reclaiming responsibility for your health. I encourage you to understand that drug therapy and disease management is an illusion. See past the illusion, and you will have found the secret to aging healthier.

While we're all going to get older, there are two paths from which to choose. I will show you the path the pharmaceutical companies don't want you to know about.

## YOUR HORMONES – CLOSE UP

In the previous chapter I provided an introduction to your hormones. Here's a closer look at testosterone, progesterone, and estrogen.

### Testosterone

While the adrenal gland produces some of the testosterone found in women, its primary source is the ovary. As you have learned in the previous chapter, women aged twenty to forty lose fifty percent of their testosterone production. Symptoms of low testosterone may include "brain fog," loss of memory focus and concentration, fatigue, insomnia, and loss of sex drive. Women may experience irritability, anxiety, depression, night sweats, joint pains, and weight gain, especially across the mid-section (belly fat). This can occur even if you are following an exercise regime and following the direction of the newest fad diet on the market.

Testosterone begins to decrease earlier than the other ovarian hormones. Many women do not realize that low testosterone can increase their risk for Alzheimer's disease, heart disease, breast cancer, osteoporosis, and diabetes. The benefits of bio-identical testosterone are many: improved energy, memory, focus, concentration, and sleep (which, by the way, can improve the choices we make in our eating); enhanced libido or sex drive; and reduced anxiety, irritability, and depression. (Yes, you could possibly get off those anti-depressants.) Women may also experience reduced night sweats, improvement in muscle aches and joint pains, and weight gain, even if you may be following your exercise. Balancing your testosterone with bio-identical testosterone will reduce your cholesterol and triglycerides, allowing you to avoid the side-effect-riddled statins. It will improve bone mineral density and reduce hip fractures, and can reduce your risk of Alzheimer's disease. There is very new information that suggests your risk of breast cancer will be reduced.

Without looking at their patients' lab work, most physicians tend to treat the symptoms of low testosterone in women with antidepressants, diet pills, sleeping pills, pills to improve memory, or tranquilizers. We saw that in the story of Carol and Anne. Using bio-identical hormones that mimic the testosterone made in a woman's ovaries can be a better choice for both short-term symptom relief and long-term protection of the brain, heart, breasts, and bones.

Why doesn't Big Pharma cash in on bio-identical hormone replacement? For two very significant reasons: patents and profits.

Pharmaceutical companies are not willing to support bio-identical testosterone replacement because they cannot patent a bio-identical substance. Instead, they chose to make a synthetic testosterone paired with an oral synthetic estrogen called Estratest. Unfortunately, the synthetic testosterone was poorly absorbed from the GI tract, and women never received the benefits of having their testosterone balanced.

There is no natural testosterone that is absorbed by ingesting it orally. Therefore, bio-identical testosterone hormone replacement must be given sublingually, or topically in a cream base, or by subcutaneous hormone "pellets," which are actually very tiny—about the size of a grain of rice.

The sublingual troches are very expensive, give high spikes in testosterone, and have not been shown to give long-term benefits.

The topical creams have very erratic absorptions. That means a woman's testosterone levels are unpredictable and often excessively high. In addition, because the cream must be applied daily, patient compliance is a key factor, not to mention that creams are transferable and blood levels shoot up and down like a roller coaster. There have been no studies showing long-term protection of a women's brain, bones, breasts, or heart using this delivery method.

In contrast, subcutaneous hormone pellets give women predictable testosterone levels in the desired range, twenty-four hours a day, seven days a week. These levels remain relatively constant for four to five months. I will discuss the short- and long-term benefits to this delivery method in a subsequent chapter wholly devoted to pellet therapy.

**Progesterone**
Progesterone is a hormone that is produced in the ovaries and adrenal glands. Premenopausal women need progesterone to mature the lining of the uterus in preparation for the fertilized egg for implantation. In this book, I want to limit our discussion to the value of progesterone to post-menopausal women. In women who have a uterus, progesterone prevents estrogen from over-stimulating the endometrium (the lining of the uterus). This helps protect women from endometrial cancer and from resuming their menstrual periods. This hormone also has many other benefits including improvement in mood swings, enhancing sleep, and protection against breast cancer. It works in conjunction with estrogen to protect the nerves in the brain, and thus helps women lower their risk of Alzheimer's disease.

Everyone reading this book needs to understand that these benefits are derived from using natural *bio-identical* progesterone.

Unfortunately, the synthetic progesterones known as *progestins* have very different effects in a woman's body. How did we come to use synthetic progestins instead of the bio-identical progesterone? It started as a problem of absorption. Progesterone was not able to be absorbed well orally. Physicians began using Upjohn's synthetic progestin Provera to control excess vaginal bleeding in women who had been taking only estrogen for hormonal support. Then the pharmaceutical company Wyeth-Ayerst combined this synthetic progestin with its synthetic estrogen Premarin to make the drug everyone knows as Prempro. This synthetic progestin is known to cause cancer, and it's been banned in most European countries for over fifty years.

The synthetic progestins undo the protective effect of estrogen on the heart and the brain. In an article in the *Proceedings National Academy of Science* in September 2003, the protective effect of estrogen on the nerve cells in the brain was blocked by taking the synthetic progestin (MPA). Synthetic progestins attenuate the beneficial effects that bio-identical estrogen has on your lipid profile. The most important lipid for heart protection gets *reduced* with synthetic progestins and *increased* with bio-identical progesterone.

The synthetics also increase vaso-spasm in the coronary arteries, whereas the bio-identical progesterone increases blood flow to the heart. They increase the risk of breast cancer. This was demonstrated in the Women's Health Initiate, and led to the study being stopped prematurely. The side effects of synthetic progestins—including weight gain, swelling, abdominal bloating, muscle aches, and mood disorders—make them poorly tolerated in nearly half of patients who have tried them.

Often, things happen at the same time, and the benefits of one are overshadowed by the other event. In 1998, the U.S. Food and Drug Administration approved a drug called Prometrium. A bio-identical progesterone, it was special because through the process of micronization (making the drug particles smaller), they found a way to get natural bio-identical progesterone absorbed orally.

It can also be compounded to the clinician's specifications in pills, creams, and gels. Unfortunately, the Women's Health Initiative had started its one-billion-dollar study using PremPro. The benefits of the natural hormone were overshadowed by the devastating side effects of PremPro reported in the *Journal of the American Medical Association* in July 2002. Women were stopping their hormone replacement at an exponential rate when hey should have been using the safer and more beneficial natural progesterone.

It is amazing and ludicrous that the PhRMA-supported FDA has not recalled PremPro from the shelves to help protect women everywhere. The bottom line is women deserve to have hormone replacement with the specific hormone in which their body is deficient. Just like with testosterone, and as you will see with estrogen, we have the natural bio-identical progesterone. Don't accept anything else. In a study in the *Journal of Women's Health & Gender-Based Medicine* in May 2000, when compared to synthetic progesterone (*medroxyprogesterone acetate*), micronized bio-identical progesterone offered the best potential for improving quality of life and improvement of menopausal symptoms. The same conclusion was reached by Dr. Fitzpatrick and his team at the Mayo Clinic, as reported in the Mayo Clinic *Women's Healthsource* in August 1999.

## Estrogen

The final hormone to disappear as a woman reaches menopause is estrogen. Estrogen protects against osteoporosis, Alzheimer's disease, colon cancer, strokes, heart disease, and macular degeneration. Estrogen deficiency results in vulvovaginal atrophy, incontinence, increased wrinkles on face, decreasing collagen leading to sagging skin on face, fatigue, depression, mood swings, and decreased sex drive. Women understand that they feel better with estrogen than without it. They understand that to age healthier, look younger, and feel their best, they need estrogen.

In women, the ovaries produce estrogen. Approaching menopause, estrogen levels decrease by as much as eighty percent. This drop can lead to "hot flashes," vaginal dryness, and problems with urination and incontinence. While these are the most talked about symptoms, in the female body estrogen has over four hundred functions.

After age forty, a woman's progesterone production may have decreased by eighty percent. This drop in progesterone during perimenopause can lead to estrogen dominance with excess bleeding, menstrual, irregularities and mood swings.

The most important of the three estrogen hormones in the pre-menopausal years is estradiol; estrone and estriol are much less important. That is why when we replace women's waning hormones, we replace estrogen loss with estradiol.

So how did the estrogen controversy ignite, and why as physicians have we not ended the "war" over whether estrogen is good or bad? History will help us with this problem. Estrogen was first discovered in the 1930s. In fact, research on subcutaneous hormone pellet therapy also began in the 1930s using estradiol pellets in women undergoing hysterectomy. Unfortunately, the pharmaceutical industry rushed in with its patented candidate for therapy, Premarin, which was conjugated equine estrogen made from the urine of pregnant horses. In 1966 a physician named Robert Wilson wrote *Feminine Forever*, a book that endorsed Premarin, and women everyone wanted this miracle drug to maintain their femininity. Instead of promoting the safer, less expensive natural hormone estradiol, which was bio-identical to a women's ovarian estradiol, commercial interests won out. In other words, *profits* were more important than the health of the patient.

Dr. Joel T. Hargrove, director of the Vanderbilt Menopause Center, Vanderbilt University, demonstrated that natural bio-identical hormones produced better outcomes with fewer side effects than synthetic hormones. He famously said that "natural" should refer to the "structure of the hormone itself, not the source of the hormone. Premarin is a natural hormone if your native food is hay!" In addition, he found that bio-identical hormones

75

produced better patient compliance. That is an important ingredient for long-term healthy aging.

To make matters worse, as female patients began bleeding profusely, the same pharmaceutical company added a synthetic progesterone known as *medroxyprogesterone acetate* (MPA). Over time, Premarin and Prempro became two of the bestselling drugs. "Blockbuster" is the term used by the pharmaceutical industry for such drugs that rack up huge profits.

There was great consternation regarding blood clots, heart attacks, strokes, and breast cancer from using the two synthetic hormone replacement drugs. So much controversy arose that a group of physicians felt it necessary to spend one billion of your tax dollars to look at these drugs. It is unfortunate for the hundreds of millions of women who benefit from estrogen replacement therapy that no other drugs were evaluated, no other delivery methods were evaluated, no blood levels were evaluated to test balance and optimization, and no natural estradiol products that had been around for over sixty years were even considered.

In the estrogen-only arm (Premarin), there was no increase in risk of breast cancer; in fact, there was a reduction in breast cancer by approximately twenty-five percent. There was, however, increased risk of blood clots, heart attacks, and stroke. The combination of equine estrogen and MPA was covered under the progesterone section. Had these "scientists" considered other natural hormones delivered transdermally or by subcutaneous pellet placement, there would be no increase in blood clots heart or stroke.

The ramifications from this clinical oversight were devastating. In July 2002, on the heels of the Women's Health Initiative data being reported, a *TIME* magazine cover proclaimed "Hormone replacement therapy is riskier than advertised. What's a woman to do?" In less than two years, half of the women who were using systemic hormone therapy stopped the treatment. Compared with 2001, use of oral estrogen-only among women aged 50-59 years with no uterus dropped by almost 60% in 2004, 71% by

2006, and 79% in 2010 and 2011, the authors noted an article published in *Journal of the American Medical Association* in 2011.

Why is this sensationalism a problem? Because women who suffer from estrogen deprivation are likely to suffer from depression and poor quality of life, bone loss, heart disease, dementia, parkinsonism, and all-cause mortality. It was the Women's Health Initiative that got women inappropriately scared.

Analysis of the 2011 WHI-ET (Women's Health Initiative Estrogen-Alone Trial) data, done by a group at Yale University and published in the *American Journal of Public Health* in 2013, showed that a minimum of 18,600 and as many as 91,600 excess deaths occurred between 2002 and 2011 among women aged 50-59 years – who had sustained a hysterectomy due to estrogen therapy avoidance.

An earlier study in the *New England Journal of Medicine* by Dr. Hu showed a 31% decline in coronary artery disease in over 85,000 patients on HRT. This was in conjunction with a 175% increase in the use of HRT. Then two years later, the WHI destroyed the great progress we were making in healthy aging for women.

It is up to physicians to stay up-to-date on the real benefits of estrogen replacement therapy. Too few patients who are estrogen deficient are on ERT. Many physicians are afraid to give prescriptions for it, and mislead patients as to the real benefits and few side effects.

More than fifty percent of women discontinue ERT in the first year. It is paradoxical that women will take birth control pills with little fear, but have a psychological blockade when it comes to taking menopause replacement therapy with hormone doses far less than the levels found in birth control pills. It is the fault of poor education and training on the proper administration of hormones to women in all primary care fields, including

77

obstetrics and gynecology. As physicians, we must do a better job of staying up on the literature, do a better job of seeing through the 'smoke and mirrors' created by sensationalized studies of little substance, and do a better job of helping our patients age healthier.

## TAKING BIO-IDENTICAL ESTROGEN

I want women to know that natural bio-identical estrogens are very safe and very effective as alternatives to synthetic estrogen. They are even safer when not taken orally. Oral estradiol creates a large spike in estradiol levels in the bloodstream. The levels, however, are relatively short lived, and the women are left with the side effects of fluid retention, breast tenderness, vaginal bleeding, and headaches. As the estradiol levels fall, symptoms return before the next dose is due.

There are patches of pure bio-identical estradiol. In eighty-five percent of patients they will help reduce "hot flashes" successfully. In my experience they work well, without increasing risk of blood clots; however, nearly half of patients don't absorb the estradiol adequately. Your physician should be checking your hormones to assure adequate optimization.

You may also choose to use a cream or gel. Many "anti-aging" clinics prescribe Bi-EST Cream. It is a combination of estradiol and estriol. This product must be used twice a day, and does not achieve adequate estradiol levels in the bloodstream. The expense doesn't produce the desired outcome, there are no protective effects, and patient compliance is poor. Estrasorb is another prescription cream. It has reasonable absorption and will reduce hot flashes in most; however, the estradiol levels do not remain constant and are not adequate for brain, heart, and bone protection. Also, in my experience most patients stop this form of therapy within the first year.

I am often asked about herbal preparations from health food stores. These include the phytoestrogens and black cohash. I do not recommend patients using them, because they are only minimally effective for menopausal symptoms. On a long-term basis they confer no bone, brain or heart protection.

The best option is subcutaneous pellet hormone therapy. These tiny pellets—each is about the size of a grain of rice—are made of pure bio-identical estradiol. They are placed painlessly beneath the skin of the hip, and generally two or three insertions a year give you consistent estradiol levels without the spikes seen with oral therapy and with minimal side effects. My patients have found this method so attractive that 96% stay on them for a minimum of three years. Even more important, 95% get symptom relief of their "hot flashes" and vaginal dryness within first few weeks of therapy.

As I have stated before, I have devoted the majority of my professional career managing women's health. With the help of many patients throughout the years of delivering their babies and then following their health concerns into the "season" of the perimenopause, and hearing thousands of cries for help, I have devoted the last decade to finding those answers.

Later in the book, I'll reveal more about this method in the chapter devoted strictly to pellet therapy.

# CHAPTER 5

# NATURAL HORMONE REPLACEMENT FOR MEN

While the casual observer may assume that bio-identical hormone replacement is something that is strictly for women, the truth is very different. Many men need hormone replacement too.

I speak from personal experience. For the early part of my life I never really believed in male menopause, also known as andropause. Like most men, I was ill-informed when the time approached, and perhaps a bit in denial. It was very evident that my female patients were experiencing this change, but we are the hunters, the stronger of the sexes; this was just normal gradual aging, wasn't it?

In my early forties, I knew I was getting older, and my body and mind began changing. I was getting sleep deprived, my sexual performance was declining, and the urge to hit the gym was no longer a priority. Late nights and early mornings delivering babies was exhausting. Work wasn't enjoyable anymore; it was irritating. My workouts were much less productive. I was developing belly fat. My cholesterol was on the rise. Trying to remember things that were once a snap now seem to take forever.

Despite the obvious signs, entering into the "season" of andropause was not a consideration. Unlike women, we really don't talk about our aging bodies. However, after hearing years of symptoms and concerns from our talkative counterparts, although each unique, the underlying chief complaints were drawing a very straight and narrow line. Knowing that they were experiencing real hormonal changes, how are we any different?

Once I opened up to the possibility my testosterone could be low, that my symptoms were not permanent, and that my mind and body could be rejuvenated, I sought out the solution.

## WHAT TESTOSTERONE IS
## AND WHAT IT DOES

Of all the human hormones, testosterone is wrapped in the most myth and mystery. Many men—and women—simply see it as the "sex hormone" that gives men their sex drive. In this simplistic belief, high testosterone equals high sex drive. Low testosterone equals poor bedroom performance.

Of course, this image of testosterone as being the he-man hormone is a vast oversimplification. Before we discuss the complex ways in which testosterone levels affect the minds and bodies of men, let's make sure that we know what this stuff is, where it comes from, and what it does in your body.

Found in mammals, reptiles, birds, and other vertebrates, testosterone is a steroid hormone from the androgen group. Steroid hormones help control metabolism, inflammation, immune functions, development of sexual characteristics, and the ability to withstand illness and injury—hence the popular use of the term "steroids" for the stuff that athletes inject. In male mammals, testosterone is secreted primarily by the testicles, although small amounts are also secreted by the adrenal glands.

In men, testosterone aids in the development of male reproductive organs such as the testes and prostate, and promotes secondary sexual characteristics including the growth of body hair and increased muscle and bone mass.

Males produce more than females; on average, in adult males, levels of testosterone are eight times as great as in adult females.

When the higher rate of metabolic *consumption* of testosterone in males is taken into account, the actual daily production of testosterone is about twenty times greater in men than in women.

Testosterone levels can be measured by a simple blood test. In males, the first physical signs of increased testosterone are apparent during puberty. A boy's voice changes, his shoulders broaden, and his facial structure becomes more masculine. Testosterone levels are at their highest during adolescence and early adulthood. The normal range of testosterone levels in healthy males is between 800 and 1,200 nanograms per deciliter (ng/dL). After age thirty, testosterone levels in men decline— sometimes precipitously.

### The History of Testosterone Therapy

Over the centuries, medical researchers have been keen to uncover the secret to male sexual function—how it began in puberty and why it seemed to wane as men reached middle age and later. After all, reproduction is a key mystery of life, and if you could unlock its secrets the effects on human life could be profound.

The history of testosterone therapy has, and continues to, resemble a mystery novel. There has long been intrigue and controversy. Some of the first experiments involving testosterone were conducted on chickens. In 1767, John Hunter transplanted testes from roosters into the abdomen of a hen. While the testes adhered to the hen's intestine, they produced no noticeable change in the hen.

In 1849, Arnold A. Berthold tried a similar experiment but with a twist. Of six roosters, two were used as a control group, two were castrated but had their testes transplanted back into their own bodies at a distant location, and the remaining two were castrated and left to develop with no testes. Unsurprisingly, Berthold found that the two castrated chickens never developed adult male characteristics. However, the two chickens with the transplanted testes developed into mature adult roosters. This suggested that the location of the organ was not crucial to how these internal secretions worked; the secretions must travel freely through the bloodstream.

In 1889, Harvard University professor Charles Edouard Brown-Séquard contributed an article in the *London Lancet* entitled, "The Effects Produced on Man by Subcutaneous Injections of a Liquid Obtained From the Testicles of Animals." He wrote, "There is no need of describing at length the great effects produced on the organization of man by castration, when it is made before the adult age. It is particularly well known that eunuchs are characterized by their general debility and their lack of intellectual and physical activity…. It is known that well-organized men, especially from twenty to thirty-five years of age, who remain absolutely free from sexual intercourse or any other causes of expenditure of seminal fluid, are in a state of excitement, giving them a great, although abnormal, physical and mental activity. These two series of facts contribute to show what great dynamogenic power is possessed by some substance or substances which our blood owes to the testicles. For a great many years I have believed that the weakness of old men depended on two causes—a natural series of organic changes and the gradually diminishing action of the spermatic glands."

His article throws into perfect relief the three most persistent beliefs that people have had about testosterone (the "Elixir of Life"): that lack of it makes a young man weak; that if a man "saves it" by celibacy he will become stronger; and that the decline of old age is due to a loss of the magical elixir.

Of the first belief I'll reserve judgment, and the second we now know is laughable. But the third is no laughing matter to millions of men as they open that invitation to join AARP for the first time.

Brown-Séquard injected testicular extract into himself, and then claimed amazing physical and mental improvements. Of course there was no proof that it worked, and it was later discovered it was merely a placebo effect. No matter! By the end of 1889, more than 12,000 physicians were selling the "Elixir of Life" throughout Europe and North America.

The idea that some mysterious substance in animal testicles could offer performance-enhancing benefits in athletes has been firmly planted in the research community ever since 1896, when Austrian physiologist Oskar Zoth published a paper in which he hypothesized that injections of steroid-based testicular extracts could enhance athletic performance. He somewhat presciently wrote, "The training of our athletes offers an opportunity for further research and a practical assessment of our experimental results."

In the 1920s came our next testosterone pioneer, Eugene Steinach, a Viennese physiologist, who invented the "Steinach operation" (or "Steinach vasoligature"), the goals of which were to reduce fatigue and the consequences of aging, and to increase overall vigor and sexual potency in men. It consisted of a half- (unilateral) vasectomy, which would cause the sperm-producing tissue to back up and atrophy, making more room for the interstitial or Leydig cells that are also produced in the testicles, which would then flood the bloodstream with hormones and new energy. He trained numerous surgeons in the art of "Steinaching" eager patients. In the Roaring Twenties, thousands of Steinach operations were performed in the US and around the world, from Chile to India.

Any apparent results were a placebo effect. The biological ideas that underlay Steinaching have long been discredited; a vasectomy doesn't stimulate the overproduction of Leydig cells, as Steinach supposed.

Steinach was followed by a Swiss genitourinary surgeon, Paul Niehans, who ingeniously transferred live testicular cells to increase "testicular secretions." But what were these "secretions"? What was helping these "middle-aged, listless individuals"?

In 1935, researchers K.G. David, E. Dingemanse, J. Freud and E. Laqueur, who were backed by the Organon Pharmaceutical Company in Oss, The Netherlands, published the now classic paper "*Über krystallinisches mannliches Hormon aus Hoden*

*(Testosteron) wirksamer als aus harn oder aus Cholesterin bereitetes Androsteron,*" or, "On crystalline male hormone from testicles (testosterone) effective as from urine or from cholesterol." They named the hormone "testosterone" from the stems of "testicle" and "sterol," and the suffix of "ketone."

Thanks to the breakthrough by Organon, the testosterone industry was born. The synthesis of testosterone came later by Leopold Ruzicka, and the researchers applied for a patent. In 1939, Ruzicka shared the Nobel Prize for chemistry with Adolf Friedrich Johann Butenandt, another researcher in the field of human hormones.

These great pioneers from all parts of the world had discovered the "secretion." Since then, the question has been who to treat, with which problems, with how much testosterone, and whether should it be bio-identical or synthetic.

In 1945, Paul Henry de Kruif, an American biologist, wrote a book on testosterone, *The Male Hormone*. There were a number of studies in the "golden age of steroids" from 1940-1960. They mostly were haphazard, using synthetic injections or oral methyl testosterone. In California, bodybuilders experimented with testosterone and helped develop the multi-million-dollar black market in testosterone supplements that flourishes today.

In 1966, a physician named Robert Wilson wrote *Feminine Forever*, which was the stimulus for women to start getting their hormones replaced. This book sparked discussions about testosterone replacement in men. The products were "synthetic" testosterone compounds, and without guidance as to dosing, a number of males became aggressive, blaming testosterone, and its use quickly diminished. In the 1980s, the World Health Organization performed a study to see if anabolic steroids could be used as a male contraceptive. The results were very efficacious and with minimal side effects. It is interesting and perplexing that the doses used for contraception in the male exceed those used by Olympic sprinter Ben Johnson for which he was banned from the Olympics. It wasn't until the new millennium that testosterone was re-evaluated as a "healthy aging" drug.

## THE MODERN TESTOSTERONE INDUSTRY

Today, physicians write more than seven million prescriptions per year for testosterone products. It's a two-billion-dollar-a-year business for the pharmaceutical industry—a "blockbuster" for sure.

The pioneers have given way to big pharmaceutical companies vying for that two-billion-dollar gold mine. Meanwhile, the black market for anabolic steroids has staked its claim. It has found its way into modern houses, where men self-diagnose and administer this dangerous drug, all trying to stay ahead of the inevitable aging process. This has caused men to suffer horrendous side effects including aggression, heart disease, and testicular atrophy. Major sports athletes from pro football, cycling, baseball and bodybuilding have fallen from fame and have had their careers tarnished permanently.

As with all great mysteries, there must be a problem to solve. What is the right drug, at the right dose, given by the best route of administration? Where is our solution? Is it synthetic or bio-identical? Where is the hero who actually wants to improve the health and vitality of men as they age, rather than sell out to commercial profiteering? This book and this chapter help solve the mystery of hundreds of years.

### Age and Testosterone

Male andropause can begin any time after age thirty-five. It has also been termed androgen deficiency in the adult male (ADAM). Each year thereafter, men lose between one and five percent of their testosterone production. That means on average men lose twenty percent of their testosterone per decade. Many men lose it much more quickly.

In conjunction with this *decrease* in testosterone as we age, there is an *increase* in sex hormone binding globulin (SHBG), the protein that binds up our useable testosterone (T). So we make less T, and more of it gets sucked up like a sponge by the SHBG. Unlike female menopause, which occurs more as an event or rapid loss of hormone production, the "season" of andropause can be indolent, and therefore harder to pinpoint, in its onset. Aging in males, like females, is multi-factorial. Some men have great genes and long-lasting hormone balance. Others have genetic alterations, stressful lives, sub-optimal immune systems, and early hormone imbalances leading to accelerated, unhealthy aging.

The symptoms are an easy way to help make the diagnosis. Men feel fatigued (especially after noon), experience insomnia, and have decreased memory, focus, and concentration. They have "presenteeism," where they go to work and they are present and accounted for, but their performance is sub-par. Workouts are less productive, and in fact they begin losing muscle mass. Sexual performance is decreased. This is most noticeable by a loss of morning erections and loss of erections after ejaculation. Some men even lose their libido. These symptoms have deleterious effects on a man's relationship with his partner. It is by no coincidence that the peak years for divorce correspond to the early years of andropause.

Over the long term, men with low testosterone have an increased risk for heart disease, stroke, diabetes mellitus, Alzheimer's disease, prostate cancer, arthritis, osteoporosis and fractures, and sarcopenia (muscle loss).

## Testosterone Replacement Choices

What responsible and safe steps can males entering andropause take to protect their bodies and minds?

There are a number of choices—many of them questionable and unstudied. Because men produce twenty times more testosterone daily compared to woman, men require obviously higher doses to treat their symptoms and for long-term prevention of the diseases listed above.

- Anabolic steroids that cannot be metabolized to estrogen are not part of a healthy aging plan. They have deleterious side effects, including aggression, and can damage the heart, liver and kidneys.

- The creams and gels commercialized by the pharmaceutical companies, albeit bio-identical, have erratic absorption, and do not achieve blood levels adequate to treat the symptoms of low testosterone. They certainly are not capable of preventing heart disease, Alzheimer's disease, diabetes, or osteoporosis. They are, however, a great example of the commercialization of medicine and the lack of concern by pharmaceutical companies for treating the aging male with something that might make them healthier, not just generate profits.

It is prudent to recall the study published in the journal *Circulation* in 2007, the official journal of the American Heart Association. They looked at more than 11,000 men between the ages of forty and seventy-nine. The levels of testosterone before therapy, if low, had increased risk of heart disease, cancer, and all causes of death. Based on this study and numerous others, it is prudent to achieve higher levels of testosterone similar to those seen in our twenties.

As of this writing, a growing number of men throughout the United States are pursuing potential AndroGel lawsuits, Testim lawsuits, Axiron lawsuits, and other testosterone drug lawsuits. All of the complaints filed in state and federal courts nationwide involve similar allegations that men suffered heart attacks, strokes, blood clots or other serious and sometimes fatal injuries as a result of heart problems from Androgel and other testosterone drugs, and that inadequate warnings have been provided to men and the medical community.

- Synthetic injections including testosterone cypionate, testosterone enanthate, and the new longer-acting testosterone undecanoate.

The first two, testosterone cypionate and testosterone enanthate, must be administered at least weekly, if not twice a week. This could require 104 shots per year per patient. In my experience, this leads to a compliance problem, and men simply will not stay on the therapy. These products are also produced in an oil base, typically cottonseed oil. This allows for a "time release" of the synthetic testosterone, which then must go to the liver for conversion to the active compound testosterone. Many men have experienced allergies to the cottonseed oil and have developed scar tissue from the oil at the injection sites. Even though cypionate and enanthate can achieve successful blood levels, there is a "roller coaster" effect with blood levels going up and down on a weekly basis. Additional problems from these two medications include: a lowering of the HDL cholesterol levels (good cholesterol), an excessive increase in red blood cells, and—most disturbing—an increase of a substance from our platelets called thromboxane A2. This substance has been associated with increasing platelet "stickiness" and constriction of blood vessels. It is not known but surmised that this may lead to increase in heart attacks in the elderly, especially if they have pre-existing heart disease.

The final drug in this category is testosterone undecanoate. It has been recently approved by the FDA for the treatment of hypogonadism in males. It is a "synthetic" and has all the pitfalls described for the other injectable testosterone preparations. It also has two additional issues. Most importantly, patients have had pulmonary oil micro-embolisms. This where small oil droplets have travelled to the lung and caused fatalities. There has also been anaphylactic reactions to the oil. Currently, AVEED, as the product is known as, is only available on a restricted program.

- The final, and best choice is treatment with subcutaneous hormone pellets. While I'll present an entire chapter devoted to this therapy, here's an overview. Each testosterone "pellet" is tiny—only about the size of a grain of rice. As in the female, it is implanted painlessly beneath the skin in the buttock or sometimes the abdomen.

The pellets are natural bio-identical testosterone. Their benefits are many and side effects few. Most important, they maintain relatively constant blood levels, avoiding the "roller coaster" effect of injections and creams. They also achieve adequate blood levels to be beneficial to the symptoms of low testosterone, and more importantly are a great proactive step to avoiding the serious maladies that await us in each decade as we get older. This therapy is made even more fascinating because men only have to receive the therapy usually twice a year. They are therefore the *sine qua non* needed for "healthy aging."

## MALE ESTROGEN

Rather than cover estrogen in men in a separate section, its ties to testosterone are integrally related, and therefore I'll cover the key points men need to know here. While most men think of estrogen as a hormone found only in females, nothing could be further from the truth. Men need estrogen. Testosterone raises estradiol levels via an enzyme called aromatase. Everybody has a different amount of this enzyme, and therefore our estradiol levels vary from person to person. There is an "ideal range" your doctor should try to maintain.

The pharmaceutical and neutraceutical companies are flagrant in their propaganda that estrogen is bad for the heart, bad for the prostate, will cause you to gain "belly fat," and increase your risk for prostate cancer. There is no evidence to support these claims. They want you to buy Arimidex, Femara, and Chrysin, to name just a few. They even are teaching amateur "anti-aging" doctors to use testosterone pellets with Arimidex in all their patients. This can have disastrous results!

Many of the long- and short-term benefits of testosterone are getting lost with this fundamentally flawed and medically unsubstantiated algorithm. Men have increase in heart disease, bone loss, increased risk for Alzheimer's disease, increased cholesterol, and serious aggressive behavior. If a male patient has symptoms from increased estrogen, like breast swelling or nipple sensitivity, I of course treat it with a natural aromatase inhibitor like diindolemethane (DIM), or one of the prescription medications like Arimidex or Femara.

A study conducted by researchers at Massachusetts General Hospital (MGH) and published in The New England Journal of Medicine in 2013, showed a clear link between estrogen and male health. Joel Finklestein, of the Endocrine Unit at MGH and associate professor of medicine at Harvard Medical School, said in *Medical News Today*, "This study establishes testosterone levels at which various physiological functions start to become impaired, which may help provide a rationale for determining which men should be treated with testosterone supplements…. But the biggest surprise was that some of the symptoms routinely attributed to testosterone deficiency are actually partially or almost exclusively caused by the decline in estrogens that is an inseparable result of lower testosterone levels."

The take-home lesson for men is that estrogen, like testosterone, has beneficial effects that are both short- and long-term.

## GROWTH HORMONE

Produced in the pituitary gland, growth hormone is certainly the other "fountain of youth" hormone. It is actually one of the most abundant hormones produced by the pituitary. From age twenty-one to forty, our production of GH decreases by more than fifty percent, and the exponential decline continues as we get older.

There is good news—we can recover our youthful levels through diet, testosterone, growth hormone-releasing stimulants, or the use of low dose growth hormone itself. In his landmark article in the *New England Journal of Medicine*, Daniel Rudman, MD, stated, "The effects of six months of human growth hormone on lean body mass and adipose tissue mass were equivalent in magnitude to the changes in twenty years of aging."

There were many additional benefits seen in this study. In 1997, Silvio Inzucchi wrote in the journal *Hospital Practice*, "Growth hormone deficiency is now formally recognized as a specific clinical syndrome, typified by decreased muscle mass, increased body fat, decreased exercise capacity, osteopenia (reduced bone mass), abnormal lipid profiles, and diminished well-being." Do these symptoms sound familiar? Do they sound like testosterone deficiency? They will also sound like thyroid deficiency in a later chapter.

The benefits from human growth hormone continue to be discovered: increase in muscle mass, loss of free fat mass, improved energy, improved immune function, better memory, and psychological well-being, enhanced sexual performance, improved bone strength, and improved lipid profile.

The mystery of aging is becoming clearer. More importantly, the pathway to healthy aging is also becoming clearer. My friend and colleague Thierry Hertoghe, a third-generation endocrinologist and world-renowned expert in anti-aging, believes testosterone and growth hormone are the medicines of the future.

It took decades to get female HRT to be accepted. It has taken more than a century to refine testosterone administration to males. Even though there continues to be numerous studies on the safety of high-frequency low-dose growth hormone, its acceptance by physicians, medical boards, and the FDA has been slow. This is sad, considering its low side effects and amazing benefits.

A great resource where you can see many of the studies and a great review on human growth hormone is the book *Grow Young with HGH*, written by Dr. Ronald Young, president of the American Academy of Anti-Aging Medicine.

Presently, growth-hormone-releasing secretagogues, which stimulate your own pituitary to produce growth hormone, are used primarily in research protocols. There is growth hormone releasing factors 2 and 6, and sermorelin available as a daily injectable to help release additional growth hormone from your own pituitary. The FDA has approved these medications for adult growth hormone deficiency. They have taken a hard stance against physicians using growth hormone, or its releasing factors, as an anti-aging therapy.

If growth hormone is indeed "a fountain of youth" hormone and men will lose significant amounts as they age, what are we to do until our federal regulatory bodies raise their awareness and support this life-changing healthy-aging medication?

Enter testosterone, the hero in the battle to maintain our growth hormone production. Curtis Hobbs and his co-workers at Madigan Army Medical Center showed that maintaining a man's testosterone level in the upper physiologic range, produced a 22% increase in IGF-1 (insulin growth factor 1), which is the marker for increased growth hormone. This was enough of an increase to put these men at a "very high functioning level." It's amazing that a free increase in our growth hormone is an additional benefit of testosterone hormone optimization. This is no small benefit, as growth hormone injections cost up to $700 per month, notwithstanding their scrutiny by regulatory boards everywhere.

For men, although the synthetic testosterone injections will achieve blood levels above the median, their side effects and long-term compliance make them a runner-up choice for testosterone deficiency. Subcutaneous hormone pellet therapy using bio-identical testosterone is the clear winner, as you'll see in the next chapter.

CHAPTER 6

# PELLET THERAPY —THE KEY TO OPTIMIZING AND BALANCING YOUR HORMONES

With well over thirty years of practicing conventional hormone replacement therapy, and after working with tens of thousands of women who wanted and needed to be rescued from their unhappy lives after the onset of perimenopause and menopause, I knew there had to be a better solution to the conventional hormone therapy that the medical establishment and the global pharmaceutical industry were offering. I didn't know it, but the answer I was looking for was right under my nose, hidden from view by the barrage of new and trendy drugs the pharmaceutical companies thought it best for me to prescribe to my patients. The bandwagon music was so loud and the blizzard of marketing so blinding that I never saw or heard of hormone pellet therapy.

One day, one patient changed my world—and hers—forever.

At age forty-one, a patient of mine named Sherri was diagnosed with fibroid tumors in her uterus. Although her tumors were benign she needed to undergo a hysterectomy. Now without her uterus, tubes, and ovaries, she was obviously hormone deficient. To treat her, I prescribed the usual cocktail of synthetic estrogen pills. Despite the treatments she remained depressed and

95

fatigued, was not sleeping well, functioned poorly at work, and was gaining weight. I fired a barrage of medications at her, from synthetic pills to bio-identical patches. She felt no better, and in fact her condition worsened over time.

At the urging of one of her friends, she saw another physician, who implanted estrogen and testosterone hormone pellets into the fat of one of her buttocks. Fortunately, Sherri did not stop coming to see me. I knew that she had received treatment elsewhere, and of course as her doctor, I wanted—and needed—to know how she was doing.

I asked her, "Well, Sherri how are you feeling now?"

She told me that within two months of beginning this new course of treatment, she was feeling amazing. Depression was gone! Weight decreasing! No hot flashes! Sleeping better! Most importantly, her marriage was resurrected and she was able to get back her original stamina at work. Sherri had regained her life and wanted me to investigate this therapy for my other patients.

*Investigate I did!*

First performed in 1939, subcutaneous hormone pellet therapy quickly became an accepted practice. In 1941, Dr. Daniel Mishell wrote in the *American Journal of Obstetrics and Gynecology* that he found hormone pellet therapy to be "a safe and simple office procedure." He stated, "During the past year, we have been gratified by the clinical results obtained with the implantation of pellets of estrone in the treatment of menopause. We found that a prolonged, continuous absorption of a small amount of hormone over a long period of time resulted from this method of therapy."

In 1949, Dr. Robert Greenblatt wrote an amazing article in the *American Journal of Obstetrics and Gynecology* on hormone pellet therapy. He began by stating that because the hormones were released on a continual basis, they more nearly reflected the physiologic action of the hormones produced by the ovary.

Think about it: If we could give a bio-identical hormone that was identical in structure to what the ovary and or testicle produced and it was given in a like manner to the ovary or testicle, we could turn back the clock to a time when our hormones were balanced.

As you know, men and women all age differently, and hormone pellet therapy has become a time-tested treatment allowing your physician to individualize your hormone optimization.

Hormone pellets are plant-based. More specifically, they are made from wild yams. The plant-based bio-identical estradiol and testosterone is converted to a powder in the United States and multiple countries around the world. Once the powder has been checked for purity and potency, it's placed under sterile conditions into a dye press. Using thousands of pounds of pressure, the powder is compressed into tiny cylinders referred to as pellets. Smaller than a grain of rice, pellets deliver consistent, healthy levels of hormones for three to four months in women and four to five months in men, which I'll review in more detail below. They avoid the fluctuations of hormone levels seen with every other method of delivery. Pellets *do not* increase the risk of blood clots like conventional or synthetic hormone replacement therapy. In 1993, Dr. Studd was one of many authors to make this claim, and no studies to date have demonstrated an increase in blood clots from hormone pellets.

Since subcutaneous hormone pellets for women and men have been available since the 1930s, their absorption has been repeatedly tested and is extremely predictable. Peak serum testosterone levels with the testosterone pellets usually occur at four weeks after implantation. Women will begin experiencing the benefits within one week and men within two weeks. Symptoms are relieved for months, avoiding having to use daily pills or creams, and weekly shots. By month four or five, testosterone levels drop to below 500 ng/dl, at which time symptoms return; this is the patient's signal that reinsertion is necessary.

Each individual has his/her own reproducible levels where they find the consistency in mood, resolution of their symptoms, and improvement in quality of life, all without painful injections. This makes pellet therapy a superior form of hormone replacement therapy.

There is also a 96% continuation rate. That continuation rate is the highest amongst all forms of treatment, and certainly benefits patients in receiving long-term protection to their brain, heart, bones, joints, and prostate. This was reported in 1997 by Dr. David Handelsman in *Clinical Endocrinology*, based on his thirteen years of treating patients and looking at the effectiveness of the therapy.

### Inserting the Pellet

A common question is this: Are the pellets surgically implanted?

No! They are placed painlessly under the skin of your buttock. A small amount of local anesthetic is used for numbing the area. To insert the pellet—which is no larger than a grain of rice—I use a patented trocar that resembles a miniature epidural needle. After insertion, a steristrip is used to close the entry point.

When you leave my office, you can go about your regular life. You can go to work and drive your car. There are just a few restrictions: For three days, no swimming, hot tubs or baths. Not to worry—showers are fine. No strenuous exercise that works the gluteal (buttock) muscles for three days. That is it!

### Patient Perspective

Rylie was a thirty-five-year-old woman scheduled for hormone pellet therapy to optimize her hormones. When she arrived at my office she was a bit nervous, which is certainly not unusual. Her girlfriend had received her pellets the month before and had explained it "was easy and did not hurt."

Rylie gave her consent and her hormone pellets were inserted in less than five minutes. She said, "That didn't hurt at all! I had worried so much and it was so easy." She went home and resumed her normal activities except for the few restrictions I mentioned above.

## PROVEN EFFECTIVENESS OF HORMONE PELLET THERAPY

In many places around the world, bio-identical hormone pellets are the standard of care for the administration of steroid hormones. Companies like BioTE Medical, LLC in Irving, Texas—of which I'm the C.E.O. and medical director—train physicians across the United States in subcutaneous hormone pellet therapy. For years, they have specifically looked at just those parameters of effectiveness, safety, dose, accuracy, purity and potency of each pellet.

Regarding effectiveness, BioTE Medical has found more than ninety percent of menopausal patients obtain relief from hot flashes and night sweats. This is consistent with what Dr. Linda Cardozo reported in the *American Journal of Obstetrics and Gynecology* in 1984. Atrophy or thinning of the vagina is also resolved in nearly ninety percent of patients. Nearly three quarters of all women receive relief from their symptoms of irritability, anxiety, and depression. Many are able to get off of their side-effect-riddled anti-depressants.

Sexual desire or libido is restored in seventy-five percent of women treated with subcutaneous testosterone pellet therapy. This has been reported by multiple physician investigators around the world.

Effectiveness can also be seen using other parameters. In 1988, in the *American Journal of Obstetrics and Gynecology*, Drs. Frank Stancyk and Rogerio Lobo from the USC School of Medicine compared bio-identical estradiol patches to sub-dermal pellets. They agreed with Dr. Mishell and Dr. Novelovitz, who independently reported in 1980 and 1987 that there were "both practical and theoretical advantages" to pellet therapy over transdermal patches. The good cholesterol (HDL) rose in half the time with hormone pellets versus the patch. Estrogen levels were "more consistent and more reproducible" than with the patch.

I have found that often the patch is poorly absorbed and the patient does not receive adequate levels of estradiol to reduce hot flashes, improve vaginal dryness, or protect their bones. In addition, as with oral therapy, the patch is hampered by patient compliance issues. As Dr. Staland reported in *Acta Scandinavia* in 1978, the bottom line for patients is that pellet therapy is superior to oral or transdermal hormone replacement therapy.

In England, subcutaneous pellet therapy is the *only* method of testosterone administration licensed for women. Symptoms return when testosterone levels drop below 80-100 ng/dl. Testosterone implants last between three and five months. Patient compliance is excellent, as women appreciate only having to undergo their pellet therapy two or three times per year.

## PELLETS COMPARED TO PILLS, SHOTS, AND GELS

Oral estrogen pills are most often synthetic and associated with multiple side effects like nausea and vomiting, weight gain, and breast tenderness, to name a few. Patients have large swings in their estrogen levels. Those patients requiring testosterone are not able to receive this life-changing hormone replacement orally. This is due to the fact there is no bio-identical testosterone that is absorbed orally. Not to mention that taking a pill can lead to compliance issues.

For males, the effectiveness is even more dramatic regarding bio-identical testosterone. Since it was first synthesized by Dr. Leopold Ruzicka and Adolf Butenandt in the 1930s, testosterone has been administered by a wide variety of modalities. Oral testosterone in bio-identical form was not absorbed and therefore was not a possible route of delivery for patient therapy. The synthetic testosterones that could be absorbed orally caused toxicity to the liver and for the most part have been abandoned, except for illicit use of anabolic steroid compounds used by some athletes.

Patients have long expressed their displeasure with shots, shots, and more shots. They commonly refuse to continue parenteral therapy ("parenteral" simply means "taken into the body in a manner other than through the digestive canal, as by intravenous or intramuscular injection") because of the pain, the inconsistent results, and the cost. The "roller coaster" ride of good days and bad has made testosterone shots a poor choice for patients.

For many years, synthetic testosterone products like testosterone enanthate and testosterone cypionate have been injected in an oil base intramuscularly. These medications are time released, which is not the physiological way a man's testicles releases testosterone throughout his life. These products have to be converted to testosterone in the liver. They have a short half-life, meaning they will not give therapeutic blood levels unless administered twice a week. Most physicians have patients take their injections *every two weeks!* Unfortunately, the men may feel good for a few days but then suffer the rebound of their symptoms as their testosterone levels fall. Painful injections, wild fluctuations in blood levels, and mood swings make this modality undesirable for long-term use.

Remember that optimal outcomes require optimization of your hormones. Optimal outcomes do not occur from the "roller coaster" ride provided by shots, creams, pills, and patches.

In an effort to capitalize on this fast-growing billion-dollar market, the newest forms of testosterone delivery are gels, creams, and underarm roll-on preparations. You cannot watch TV without being bombarded with ads for Androgel, Testim, and Axiron. They are very expensive, costing more than $500 dollars per month. Their short-term effectiveness for symptoms of fatigue, erectile dysfunction, muscle loss, and weight gain is limited. Their long-term benefits in reducing heart disease, osteoporosis, Alzheimer's disease, and prostate cancer have not been shown to be effective.

Let's take a look at one such product—AndroGel. This topical testosterone gel is marketed by AbbVie Inc., a specialty biopharmaceuticals company whose parent company is Abbott Laboratories. In 2000, the topical gel was approved for use in men with testicular damage from injury, chemotherapy, or other trauma. By 2004, AndroGel was being used off-label to counteract the symptoms of andropause—or "Low T" as it was christened by Madison Avenue in a marketing move designed to make the product sound catchy and manly. In 2011, AndroGel 1.62% was approved, as the 1% preparation was found inadequate and not therapeutic for most patients.

AndroGel stands to generate substantial revenue for AbbVie. By 2012, sales of testosterone drugs grew, reaching $2 billion. The next year, AndroGel generated more than $1.4 billion, and AbbVie spent an estimated $80 million advertising it. In fact, AndroGel commands sixty percent of the testosterone replacement therapy (TRT) market.

But storm clouds are brewing for AndroGel and the other topical gels. In September 2009, the U.S. Food and Drug Administration (FDA) ordered AbbVie to add a black box warning to the label of AndroGel. The new label warned that children who were exposed to testosterone gels might develop enlarged genitals, pubic hair, increased libido, and aggressive behavior. As of this writing, drug safety advocates are petitioning for a second black box warning. This request comes after several studies that linked the use of testosterone products to an increased risk of heart attack, especially in men over age sixty-five and men with existing heart conditions. The FDA is currently reviewing this research.

Unlike pellet therapy, which has been used safely since 1939, the "Low T" gel quickly ran into trouble as claims against it mounted. On June 26, 2014, McKenzie Lake Lawyers, LLP and Morganti Legal, P.C. filed a class action lawsuit against Abbott Laboratories Ltd., Abbott Products Inc., Abbott Products Canada Inc., and AbbVie Products LLC (collectively known as Abbott), the makers and sellers of Androgel. Since 2002—only twelve years before the lawsuit—AndroGel has been approved in Canada for use in the treatment of low-testosterone conditions associated with hypogonadism.

Use of these testosterone replacement therapies have been linked to an increased risk of suffering heart attacks, blood clots, strokes and death. The McKenzie class action claim alleges that Abbott knew or should have known of these risks and failed to warn the public. The lawsuit also claims Abbott aggressively marketed AndroGel by misleading potential users about the prevalence and symptoms of low testosterone, along with the safety and efficacy of Androgel treatment, ultimately failing to protect users from serious, life-threatening, adverse medical events.

Matthew Baer, of McKenzie Lake Lawyers, explained, "In this case, as in all of these types of cases, we are concerned about whether Canadians were adequately warned of the risks associated with using this product."

Meanwhile, in the United States the Food and Drug Administration (FDA) released an updated medical guidelines list with a new medication guide for AndroGel to include blood clots in the legs and lungs as a serious side effect of taking the topical low testosterone medication. AbbVie Inc., the makers of the low testosterone therapy drug, has also updated the official AndroGel website to include symptoms of pain, swelling or redness as signs of a blood clot in the leg and difficulty breathing or chest pain as signs of a blood clot in the lung. As the FDA makes label changes regarding blood clots, they also continue to investigate the potential cardiac risks associated with testosterone products such as AdroGel as testosterone treatment lawsuits are being filed under an industry-wide testosterone consolidation pending in the U.S. District Court, Northern District of Illinois.

As of July 15, 2014 there have been 156 testosterone treatment lawsuits pending litigation that have been filed on behalf of men who allege that they suffered from heart attack, stroke, pulmonary embolism, deep vein thrombosis and other serious side-effects from using AndroGel and other testosterone therapy drugs.

The literature on sub-cutaneous hormone pellet therapy has found no increased risk of heart attack or strokes. There have been no reports of blood clots or pulmonary embolism. Pellet therapy remains a safe alternative even for men with heart disease.

## MISGUIDED OPPOSITION FROM THE MEDICAL ESTABLISHMENT

If cynical mass marketing by big pharmaceutical companies wasn't bad enough, to further muddy the waters, both patients and doctors are often confused by false and misleading material like this statement from the American College of Obstetrics and Gynecology: "In response to recent media attention being given to so-called bio-identical hormones, the American College of Obstetricians and Gynecologists (ACOG) reiterates its position that there is no scientific evidence supporting the safety or efficacy of compounded bio-identical hormones."

Even more unfortunate is the statement by the North American Menopause Society in 2012: "The term 'bio-identical hormone therapy' is also often used to describe custom-compounded hormones that are obtained at compounding pharmacies. They are not government approved and have not been tested for effectiveness, safety, dose accuracy, or purity (absence of contaminants)."

At the Annual Meeting of the American College of Obstetrics and Gynecology in 2014, Dr Wulf Utian, past president of the North American Menopause Society, said that: "compounding pharmacies put sugar in pellets and you don't know what else."

As a patient, I know that you care deeply about the purity, potency, and sterility of any product you are putting in your body. At BioTE Medical we have had an independent lab perform purity, potency and sterility tests on subdermal pellets made at three different pharmacies across the United States. The purity is very high—within three percent of the dose prescribed by the physician. (The synthetic hormones that were recommended by Dr. Utian have between ten and thirty percent variations in purity!) There are *zero* fillers in pellets. Sterility tests were performed and met the standards for autoclaved sterility. It is unconscionable that a physician would make such a fabricated statement that reflects so poorly on the American College of Obstetrics and Gynecology, and adversely affects choices men and women need to make regarding their preventative healthcare and hormone optimization. The physicians with whom I spoke after the conference were disenchanted with Dr. Utian's remarks, as they were successfully using bio-identical hormones in their practices.

## SIDE EFFECTS OF PELLET THERAPY

No medical procedure is entirely without risk. In the case of pellet therapy, evidence suggests that within a large population of patients, the minimal side effects are far outweighed by the dramatic benefits.

Safety and proper dosage go hand in hand. The absorption of hormones from pellet therapy has been established in clinical testing for more than sixty years. That is important because if you know how a hormone is absorbed and you prescribe the proper dose, then thanks to the over eighty years of clinical testing, the side effects become predictable.

For women, the most common side effects are facial hair growth and acne. Each occurs between two and ten percent of the time. If your physician utilizes proper dosing, he or she can adjust the dosing of your estradiol and testosterone pellets to minimize these side effects. Hair thinning occurs less than one percent of the time, and is reversible and treatable. Multiple reports in the literature show no increase in blood pressure and no adverse effects on liver or blood sugar.

For men, the side effects are minimal, and may include injection site problems including infections/cellulitis, pellet extrusions, and bleeding or bruising. Infections and extrusions using proper technique are reported to be six to eight percent. In addition, with optimization of a man's testosterone, he may reduce his sperm count. (Yes, you read that correctly. An *increase* in testosterone levels can actually *decrease* your sperm count. Strange but true!) In the majority of cases, if one discontinues therapy or the dosage is decreased, sperm count rebounds once baseline testosterone levels are reached.

This side effect profile invites comparison to the more serious side effects of oral synthetic hormones, which include blood clots, heart attack, stroke, and breast cancer – if synthetic progesterone is used. Reputable companies like BioTE Medical and others teach proper dosing to their physicians, providing not only the safest method of hormone replacement, but also the superior method for hormone optimization.

The bio-identical hormones in pellets are absorbed directly into the blood stream (their absorption is based on cardiac output). With all bio-identical hormones that are constantly trickling in to your system, there's no need for the medicine to pass through the liver to be converted into a usable hormone. The hormones are ready to work as soon as they are absorbed. It is through this process that mimics the ovary or testicle that they have remained safe and have very few side effects. Testosterone and estradiol implants have the longest running safety profile, they have never been recalled by the FDA, and remain, to this day, very cost effective for the patient.

## JOYCE AND MARIO

A practical example of testosterone pellet therapy comes from one of my couples. Joyce and Mario together share the benefits of hormone optimization through subcutaneous pellet therapy. Here's their story, as told by Joyce:

"For several years I had battled migraine headaches that occurred at a certain time every month. Additionally, I had noticed a decrease in energy. I knew that I needed to exercise to get into shape, but just didn't have the energy to do so. Sex twice a week was fine with me at that time, because I just didn't have the energy or desire for more.

"Someone mentioned to me that maybe I should have my hormone levels checked. Then my sister talked to me about pellet therapy, and I thought I would try it. It was suggested that my husband try it as well.

"That was the best decision we could have made! Not only has the pellet therapy relieved my migraines, but our energy levels have increased, we are both sleeping great, our moods are more even, and best of all, our sex drive has gone through the roof! Our closeness and intimacy is better than it has ever been in almost thirty years of marriage. We both have the energy to work out and are in great shape now. Simply put, we just feel better. We wish we would have done the pellets ten years ago. I've told so many people about it that there are at least twenty people whom I personally know who are now on the pellet therapy, and they're all experiencing similar results."

## BENEFITS FOR YOU

What will hormone pellet therapy do for you? I'd like to answer that in two parts. In the short term you can expect to have improved energy, improved memory focus and concentration, reduced night sweats and hot flashes, better sleep, improved sexual performance and libido, reduced mood swings, and reduced irritability, anxiety, and depression. Your muscle aches and joint pains will be improved. You will be more successful losing weight.

Most women fear losing collagen in their skin. In 1987, Dr. Brincat reported in the journal *Obstetrics and Gynecology* that there was **no** statistical increase in collagen if patients used estradiol gel; however, when taking estradiol pellet therapy there was a statistically significant increase in a patient's collagen in multiple locations on her body. That increase in collagen was nearly forty percent.

Exercise regimens will be more productive and recovery times decreased. Long term, you will reduce your risk for heart disease, diabetes, metabolic syndrome, cancer, Alzheimer's disease, macular degeneration, rheumatoid arthritis, and osteoarthritis.

In 1990, Dr. Studd showed an 8.3% increase in bone mineral density in women taking estradiol and testosterone pellet therapy. In contrast, his colleague Dr. Anderson reported that women using estradiol patches *lost* bone density. Successful restoration of bone mineral density and reversal of osteoporosis and osteopenia has been shown in numerous other studies as well. Along with successful bone remodeling, the women experienced a reduction in hip and spine fractures.

In over eighty years, none of the studies have shown an increase risk of breast cancer, and many have shown a reduction in its incidence. In 2004, Dr. Constantine Dimitrakakis reported in *Menopause* that those patients taking bio-identical testosterone with their other hormone replacement regimen had a lower number of breast cancers.

To all the naysayers, to all the physicians who, if they are not up on something they are down on it, to all of the academic teachers in our medical schools who have shunned bio-identical hormone optimization, and to the insurance companies who believe hormone pellet therapy is experimental, the evidence of efficacy, purity, sterility, and the amazing long-term side-effect profile lend proof to the value of this therapy to men and women. Those men and women who want to age healthier, live happier, and have more productive lives should demand that their hormones be evaluated before they are randomly overmedicated for diseases they do not have. Testosterone and estrogen delivered by hormone pellet implant is the most effective healthy-aging, health-promoting, and disease-preventing treatment available. Maybe that is why ninety-seven percent of men and women continue this therapy, as opposed to the fifty percent who discontinue oral HRT after just one year.

# CHAPTER 7

# TREATING THE SILENT SCOURGE OF THYROID DISEASE

For years I saw patients who were tired, depressed, gaining weight, and experiencing joint pain. They had cold hands and poor memories, and were irritable, anxious, and moody. Like most physicians twenty or thirty years ago, I thought these patients needed anti-depressants and other "band-aid" fixes.

After I realized that these symptoms could be the result of testosterone imbalance, I began improving the lives of men and women by replacing their testosterone. But they did not always feel fully revitalized. The answer had to lie elsewhere.

There are over two hundred symptoms related to thyroid disease. It is insidious, elusive, and a great masquerader. When seeing these patients, I did not think about thyroid disease, and the lab tests that I had been taught in medical school to workup this unsuspected illness did not tell the whole story. My teachers had taught us the wrong test. It was not until I started looking at the *patients* instead of the *lab slips* that I found it easy to identify the illness that was being overlooked by many physicians.

Thyroid imbalance can not only lead to a plethora of symptoms, but it also plays a part in many diseases including cardiovascular disease, osteoporosis, obesity, diabetes, and female infertility.

Coincidentally, my colleague, Dr. Edward Lichten, a board certified obstetrician and gynecologist from Birmingham, Michigan was having the same problem. In practice for the same number of years as me, he wrote a book entitled *Textbook of Bio-identical Hormones: Guiding Health in Uncertain Times.* "It seems that every person seen in my office has thyroid disease or thyroid symptoms," he wrote.

Was this problem limited to Middle America? *Of course not!*

Dr. Neal Rouzier, a university-trained family practice and emergency medicine physician in California, was seeing the exact same problem in his area. It seemed that many of the nurses in the emergency room had the same symptoms, and when one of them received natural thyroid hormones, and her symptoms were resolved, they all wanted to be treated. It was a paradox; their "labs" (at least those labs he was taught to look at to diagnose thyroid disease) were normal, but the symptoms were omnipresent.

Both Dr. Broda Barnes, in his book *Hypothyroidism: The Unsuspected Illness* (1976), and Dr. Mark Starr, in his book *Hypothyroidism Type 2: The Epidemic* (2005, revised 2013), have been telling us for years that forty percent of the population is affected by thyroid disorder, but only ten percent are being diagnosed.

The thyroid gland is a vitally important hormonal gland. Located in the front part of the neck where your collar bones come together, the functions of this butterfly-shaped gland include the production of the thyroid hormones *triiodothyronine* (T3) and *tetraiodothyronine*, also known as thyroxine (T4).

The energy metabolism of all our cells starts with thyroid. It's not just about keeping us warm, it's about keeping all of our cells energized. In simple terms, if you want all your cells to be efficient and function rapidly in their attendant processes, they need thyroid hormone.

The endocrine system with its complex and intricate components are always firing messages back and forth. You can almost think of it like a communications command center. The multitude of messages being fired off and released, signal other messages to be fired off and released. This control center relies on this process in order for the rest of the communicators to do their jobs. If one message is read incorrectly, or perhaps not sent on time, the whole command center gets jammed up, almost like getting a constant busy signal.

When balancing and maintaining proper synergy in our hormonal therapies we have to consider the matrix of our command center. It truly begins in the hypothalamus, which is tucked deep within the center of our brains. This little powerhouse regulates breathing, blood pressure, and heart rate. It regulates body temperature and fluid balance.

Our hormonal balancing act depends on the hypothalamus for directing all other glands in our endocrine system. The thyroid is not autonomous; it clearly works in conjunction with other glands like the hypothalamus and pituitary gland.

Thyroxine is not an *active hormone*, but rather a *pro-hormone*. In the thyroid and numerous other cells throughout our body, it has to be converted to T3. This will be critically important when we look at treatment options. It is the key factor in why we have been mistreating patients and using the wrong medications. I will explain that in more detail later.

Hyperthyroidism can occur when too much thyroid hormone is produced. It is most often caused by Graves' disease or non-toxic goiter. It is rare; only one in a thousand women and three in ten thousand men get this disease. It was discovered early 1900s, even before we could measure thyroid hormones. Patient were "hot," with a rapid heartbeat and shaky hands, and they were riddled with anxiety.

Because hyperthyroidism is not caused by a deficiency of a hormone, I will not cover the subject here.

I want to focus on the more common problem of hypothyroidism, which is a deficiency disorder first reported in 1875 by physicians in London. It was often diagnosed by the patient presenting with a "thickening" or swelling of the skin, cold hands, and low basal body temperatures. Today, the symptoms are the same. Patients feel lethargic, tired, and sleepy. They have decreased memory focus and concentration. They have weight gain, yet their appetite is decreased. They are often cold. Their skin is dry and constipation is common. Females often have irregularities in their menstrual periods. Many patients feel depressed.

## THE THREE TYPES OF HYPOTHYROIDISM

Hypothyroidism can be divided into three disorders:

**Type 1 hypothyroidism**, whereby the thyroid gland does not produce enough thyroid hormone. It is easily detected by a thyroid panel blood test. This type of hypothyroidism only affects five percent of the population.

**Type 2 hypothyroidism** occurs at the cellular level. While the thyroid gland produces sufficient amounts of hormone, the body's cells are unable to utilize the hormone properly. It can be caused by thyroid receptors on the cells or in the cells being damaged and thereby not available for the thyroid hormone to bind to. This receptor problem can be inherited or can be caused by toxins in our environment. Very frequently, interaction of thyroid hormone and its target cell can be interrupted because of iodine deficiency. It's the most common cause of hypothyroidism in the United States, affecting upwards of forty percent of Americans, primarily middle-aged women, but also men and women of any age, and children. I'll discuss Type 2 hypothyroidism in detail later in this chapter.

**Type 3 hypothyroidism**, more commonly known as **Hashimoto's thyroiditis**, is a condition in which your immune system attacks your thyroid. The resulting inflammation often leads to an underactive thyroid gland.

Symptoms include weight gain, depression, mania, sensitivity to heat and cold, paresthesia, chronic fatigue, panic, bradycardia, tachycardia, congestive heart failure, high cholesterol, reactive hypoglycemia, constipation, migraines, muscle weakness, joint stiffness, menorrhagia, cramps, memory loss, vision problems, infertility, and hair loss. The laboratory work-up is the same as Type 1 and Type 2, but in addition, autoantibodies may be present against thyroid peroxidase and thyroglobulin. These are two important enzymes needed to convert the inactive T4 prohormone to the active T3 active hormone.

The other interesting nuance is that ninety percent of patients with Hashimoto's disease have gluten intolerance. Knowledge of this aids in therapy by replacing the deficient hormones as well as placing the patient on a gluten-free diet.

## FOCUS ON TYPE 2 HYPOTHYROIDISM

Understanding Type 2 hypothyroidism is relatively simple. It will help to remember from your high school biology lesson that within each cell of your body, the mitochondria make chemical energy, similar to the type of energy you get from a battery. The energy made by the mitochondria takes the form of a chemical called adenosine triphosphate, or ATP for short.

Under normal circumstances, T4 and T3 thyroid hormones increase the number and activity of mitochondria. More activity equals more energy. Think about what would happen if these little microscopic parts of the cell were genetically altered, or if the number of mitochondria in the cell were reduced. What if you had just enough thyroid hormone to be in the "normal range" on your blood test, but it was not enough to activate the mitochondria so they could function normally? That is exactly what happens in Type 2 hypothyroidism.

It is paradoxical that Type 2 hypothyroidism is a prevalent disorder that is not taught in medical schools, and thus remains elusive to mainstream physicians who rely solely on lab tests in their decision-making process. It is often not detected by the standard blood test used by physicians. The fact that this disease is inherited, pervasive, and not always identified by a blood test is worrisome. The number of people affected is expected to grow exponentially. Stress, illnesses, low testosterone, and diabetes can make this disorder worse.

## What Can Type 2 Hypothyroidism Do to Me?

Type 2 hypothyroidism affects many parts of the body. The central nervous system is affected, followed by the heart, muscles, all of the hormone-producing tissues, and the bones.

As reported by the Center for Disease Control, Alzheimer's disease is one of the top ten leading causes of death in the United States. Dr. Suzanne M. De La Monte, who in the year 2000 won the Alzheimer Research Medal, purported that Alzheimer's disease comes from decreased energy metabolism due to fewer mitochondria, and it is more prevalent in females. It is fascinating that these problems mirror those of hypothyroidism. Yet you do not see the medical community searching, finding, and aggressively treating Type 2 hypothyroidism as a prevention for Alzheimer's disease.

Remember the leading cause of death for men and women? It's cardiovascular disease. The causes of heart disease were first described over a century ago; curiously, hypothyroidism was not on the list. At that time heart disease was a minor problem, and hypothyroidism was nowhere near as prevalent as it is today. After World War ll, cardiovascular disease began its assault on men and women across the world. As a person at risk now and in the future for heart disease, you should be interested in the data on cardiovascular disease and hypothyroidism revealed in 1976 by Dr. Broda Barnes in his book, *Solved: The Riddle of Heart Attacks.* He found that in his patients, ninety percent of predicted heart attacks could be prevented if hypothyroidism were controlled.

It appears that his discovery has gone unnoticed by conventional medicine. In 2004, *Internal Medicine News* reported that hypothyroidism, even if mild, doubles your risk for coronary heart disease. It is my hope that a heart attack will not be the first sign that you have hypothyroidism. It is also my hope that the insidious symptoms of fatigue, dry skin, feeling cold, and depression will spark your physician to restore your thyroid function and not load you up with anti-depressants and other therapies that ignore the underlying problem.

More than 500,000 deaths occur every year from congestive heart failure. If one looks at the heart muscles of these patients, they are frequently interspersed with mucin, a glue-like substance that absorbs water and thickens tissue in a way that is not healthy. As a result, electrical stimulation to the heart muscle is diminished. Often patients develop irregular heartbeats, called arrhythmias. Patients can lose up to half of their cardiac output from this condition. From there the lungs and the kidneys are affected adversely. Mucin can be found in the skin, muscle, and soft tissue, which is a hallmark sign of hypothyroidism. It's better to treat this insidious disease early and avoid this consequence. Thyroid replacement is quickly becoming a first-line therapy following heart attacks and in patients with congestive heart failure.

The brain and the heart have many similarities. They both function poorly in the presence of inflammation. They both respond better to improved blood flow bringing vital nutrients. They both perform better when their cells are performing optimally because their energy production is maximized.

In patients with hypothyroidism, treatment with thyroid hormone not only improves the way the patients feel, it strengthens their immune system, reducing chronic infection and inflammation.

With thyroid hormone treatment the body produces more *adenosine triphosphate* (ATP), which is considered by biologists to be the energy currency of life. It is the high-energy molecule that stores the energy we need to do just about everything we do. It is present in the cytoplasm and nucleoplasm of every cell. Blood flow to the brain and to heart is improved. Long term protection for "healthy aging" is afforded.

As an aside, brain development of the fetus is dependent on normal thyroid function in the mother. If the mother is hypothyroid, the child's IQ can be lower and other neurologic functions can be altered.

Chronic lower respiratory disease is the fourth leading cause of death amongst Americans. What could thyroid disease, specifically hypothyroidism, have to do with lung disease? Quite a bit, as it turns out. If you are deficient in your thyroid hormones, you are more susceptible to pneumonia. Dr. Eugene Hertoghe, a world-renowned endocrinologist, reported in 1914 that patients with hypothyroidism were more susceptible to developing asthma. If you have pulmonary disease like emphysema or asthma and you want to protect your lungs from chronic infections and worsening of your breathing problems, do not neglect your thyroid.

Obesity is a major problem in the United States. Since 1985, we have seen a fourfold increase in obesity. In 2013, the American Medical Association finally classified obesity as a disease. Obesity is one of the manifestations of the metabolic syndrome. To be diagnosed with metabolic syndrome you have to have three of the five risk factors. Those include:

1. Abdominal obesity (waist measurement in males over 40 inches, and over 35 inches in females).

2. Increased triglycerides (above 150).

3. Elevated blood pressure (above 120/80).

4. Fasting blood sugar levels above 110.

5. Low HDL (good cholesterol) below 40.

Among Latin Americans there is a thirty-six percent incidence of metabolic syndrome. Both obesity and metabolic syndrome are reaching epidemic levels and both are significant risk factors for heart disease and diabetes. It is no wonder that the prevalence of diabetes increased fifty percent from 1990 to 1998. A study in *Lancet* published in August 2014 shows that forty percent of Americans will develop diabetes in their lifetime. Unfortunately, only ten percent will know they are afflicted with the disease. Years and years and years will go by, during which diabetes can ravage many of their organs.

The *Journal of the American Medical Association* reported in 2002 that forty-seven million Americans have metabolic syndrome. That number has steadily increased, not decreased.

Why are we fat? Why can't we lose weight with exercise and moderate diet? It is frustrating and often demoralizing, and many of you have just given up! The answer is that you most likely have Type 2 hypothyroidism.

Does that mean there is hope for those of you who are overweight or with metabolic syndrome? Absolutely! Keep reading.

**Meet Mary**

Mary is a forty-five-year-old patient of mine who was testosterone deficient. Despite working out and "eating healthy," she was not losing weight; in fact she was gaining weight around her midsection. She had her testosterone optimized but still could not lose weight. We knew she had hypothyroidism, but this being managed by another physician who was using synthetic thyroid hormones.

I suggested that we optimize her thyroid using Naturethroid and she agreed to try this therapy. Over the next nine months she lost fifty pounds. She continues to express her gratitude, and recently told me, "Optimizing my thyroid changed my life. My self-esteem is back and I feel better than I have in years!"

So many of the leading causes of death have their roots in untreated thyroid disease. In addition, many other ailments that affect us on a day-to-day basis also are related to thyroid deficiency. Menstrual disorders, fertility, autoimmune diseases such as lupus and rheumatoid arthritis, high cholesterol, migraine headaches, and fibromyalgia are a few that have been shown to be caused by and or worsened by hypothyroidism.

Menstrual disorders and thyroid have been linked. Dr. Broda Barnes first published on the subject in 1949. He was able to improve menstrual cramps and maintain regularity in a majority of his patients by treating them with thyroid hormone.

Modern textbooks would have you believe that fertility is not related to hypothyroidism. In my experience, a majority of infertility patients had hypothyroidism. Many had unexplained infertility and achieved pregnancy only after optimizing their thyroid hormones.

The supporting evidence linking autoimmune diseases and thyroid is intriguing. Many of the autoimmune diseases are more common in women, just as is hypothyroidism. The immune system is defective in these patients, as it is in hypothyroid patients. The connective tissue throughout the body is infiltrated with mucin in patients with autoimmune disorders. Mucin deposition is the hallmark signatory finding in hypothyroidism.

## A Patient's Perspective
Sondra was a fifty-year-old patient of mine who had developed rheumatoid arthritis. While her rheumatologist treated her with anti-inflammatory medications, I diagnosed her with testosterone, estrogen, and thyroid deficiencies. All her hormones were optimized and her quality of life was amazing. She then saw her internal medicine doctor, who performed a large battery of tests. One of these was the thyroid stimulating test (TSH), which he considered the "gold standard" in thyroid testing. Sondra's was normal and he told her to stop her thyroid hormones.

When her joint pains returned soon thereafter, she returned to me and begged me to restart her medication. I did, and once again her pain was resolved.

According to many studies, it seems more and more people are suffering from high cholesterol. As reported in an earlier chapter, an increasing number of people are taking statins. The horrific side effects from statins were also elucidated. By now you have learned that we do not suffer from statin deficiency. You also were shown that natural testosterone can lower cholesterol. Now it is thyroid's turn to right the rising cholesterol problem that is rampant in America today. People with hypothyroidism have difficulty metabolizing cholesterol through the liver to be excreted into the bowels. Dr. Lawrence Sonkin, a pioneer in endocrinology from New York, reported in the late 1970s that hypothyroid patients who received treatment with natural thyroid hormones decreased their cholesterol anywhere from twenty-five to two hundred points. This serves as a reminder of what I tell my patients: "Hormone optimization not only makes you feel good, but it's good for you."

Perhaps now it's clear that we cannot reduce cardiovascular disease until physicians awaken to see the hidden epidemic in hypothyroidism that exists in every one of their practices.

Musculoskeletal pain is no stranger to patients with hypothyroidism. It is also the hallmark symptom of fibromyalgia. The incidence of both have been paralleling one another for the past forty years. Suffice it to say that pain pills and anti-depressants are not the answer.

**Kathryn's Story**
Kathryn is a thirty-eight-year-old female who came to see me with complaints of fatigue, weight gain, muscle aches, and joint pain. She was taking *fifty-eight prescription pills a day,* including anti-depressants, narcotic pain medication, and two different anti-inflammatory prescriptions. She was feeling horrible and not getting any relief. Her marital life was in disarray and she was temporarily disabled because she could not work. Not one of the multiple physicians she was seeing—including an internist, ob-gyn, psychiatrist, and rheumatologist—had checked her hormone levels. Her testosterone was near zero and her free T3 thyroid hormone was very low. Once her hormones were optimized, I was able to wean her of all medications. She was pain free, losing weight, and said that she had not felt this good in years.

## HOW DO I FIND OUT IF I HAVE HYPOTHYROIDISM?

By now you're probably asking, "Why doesn't my doctor know about this? Why are all these people being overmedicated? Why is it difficult to find out if I am hypothyroid if I have all the symptoms?"

While interpretation of proper lab work may be helpful in making the diagnosis, symptoms and physical exams are assuredly more important, and symptom relief is most important in evaluating your therapy. Prior to 1940, clinical symptoms and basal body temperature were used to diagnose and treat hypothyroidism. Since then, it has been doctors in search of the "perfect" lab test. Unfortunately, the hunt for the perfect lab test has been a failure.

In the late 1960s, the thyroid stimulating hormone test (TSH) was introduced for commercial use. Despite being written about in multiple journals and even textbooks, there was no substantiating evidence that it was a good screening test. It seemed to be accepted by acclamation without any foundation or credible data.

The reality is TSH detects only a small fraction of people with hypothyroidism. Physicians would be more accurate and they would help more of their patients if they relied on each patient's history and physical exam. This was even validated in a great study by Dr. Peterson in the *Western Journal of Medicine* in 1992. Misinterpretation of lab work has led to overmedicating patients and not identifying their hormone deficiencies. Practically speaking, if T3 is the active thyroid hormone and the amount that is free in your blood stream is the T3 capable of binding to the cells, then would it not make sense to measure the free T3 in all patients you suspect of having hypothyroidism? Of course it would!

So for you, the important takeaway message is that forty percent of you have Type 2 hypothyroidism. You know who you are— just look at your symptoms. Conventional physicians want to rely on inaccurate lab tests creating havoc for you – the afflicted. This not only leads to missed diagnosis but increases your risk for heart disease, osteoporosis, Alzheimer's disease, fibromyalgia, and other maladies.

## Treatment

It seems that every week I have a patient who comes to my office with all the symptoms of low thyroid. I have usually already balanced their other hormones. When I suggest they have hypothyroidism, they say, "My other doctor checked my levels and they were normal."

I ask them, "Do you want to feel better, and stop feeling lousy?"

"Yes!" is the resounding answer.

It is paradoxical that patients know they have the disorder and the doctor can confirm the signs during a physical exam, but the standard lab test does not concur—and so the appropriate treatment is not given.

As inexpensive as thyroid hormone is to buy, you would think the pharmaceutical companies would want to play in this profitable sandbox. Unfortunately, they have not, and they continue to confuse physicians everywhere. In 1960, dessicated porcine thyroid (i.e., armour thyroid) lost its popularity as pharmaceutical companies began mass producing the inactive T4 hormone under the names Levothyroxine, Synthroid, and Levoxyl. Synthroid and Levothyroxine have had multiple problems with subpotency (not having the correct amount of hormone ) in their tablets.

In his amazing book *Hypothyroidism Type 2: The Epidemic*, Dr. Mark Starr referred to the principles of therapy developed by Dr. Broda Barnes, a pioneer in thyroid research, who devoted his life to the advancement of treatment in thyroid diseases. His Research Foundation, after treating thousands of patients for many years, was emphatic that desiccated thyroid is more efficacious than synthetic T4. This was again validated by Drs. Hertoghe, Baisier, and Eeckhaut in *The Journal of Nutritional and Environmental Medicine* in 2001. Patients who were taking T4 were compared to patients with hypothyroidism who were taking no medication. In the end, there was no difference in symptom relief. The patients were then given dessicated thyroid, and there was significant improvement in fatigue, cold, joint pain, depression, muscle aches, and many other symptoms. Why would anyone utilize synthetic thyroid hormones?

I have treated thousands of patients who were on synthetic thyroid hormones. In most cases their endocrinologists or primary care physicians were constantly moving the dose up and down and up and down, but the patients were feeling no better. Then they would add in a synthetic T3 hormone known as Cytomel. The problem with Cytomel is it has a very short half-life and is there and gone within hours.

Round and round these uninformed physicians went, chasing that perfect lab test. But blind devotion to lab tests will not improve the quality of anyone's life. Unfortunately, these physicians should have been striving for improvement of symptoms and a better quality of life.

The majority of my patients prefer, even demand, to be on desiccated thyroid like Armour Thyroid, Nature-Throid, or Westhroid. Their experiences, like mine and Drs. Barnes and Starr, is that desiccated thyroid is more efficacious than synthetic thyroid hormone. More important, if it makes the patient feel better, they are much more likely to continue the therapy and experience the long term benefits.

If people have religious objections to the porcine dessicated thyroid, bovine desiccated thyroid can be compounded, and it is very reasonably priced.

For those patients who are hypothyroid and are producing autoantibodies to their thyroid gland (Hashimoto's thyroiditis), the treatment remains the same, utilizing desiccated thyroid. In addition, these patients are put on a gluten-free diet. Their autoantibodies decrease and they feel incredibly better.

## Tammy Has Hashimoto's

Tammy is a forty-five-year-old female who has testosterone deficiency. She had been successfully treated with testosterone pellet therapy. Although she felt better, she continued to have chronic constipation and dry skin. She also noticed her abdomen was bloated after most meals. Her thyroid work-up revealed she had a thyroid hormone deficiency and antibodies to the enzyme in her thyroid, indicating she had Hashimoto's thyroiditis. Although she optimized her thyroid by starting Nature-Throid and iodine therapy, she had not accepted that she was gluten intolerant—the cause of the bloating and associated abdominal pain. She underwent a colonoscopy and was found to have diverticulitis with marked inflammation of the colon. This time she began the gluten-free diet and her symptoms were much improved.

Hormones always need co-factors to work. These are usually Vitamins and minerals that help the hormones achieve their desired effects in the cell. Thyroid hormone is no different. Often iodine and selenium are necessary additions to optimal therapy. As such they will be covered in the next chapter on nutraceuticals.

# CHAPTER 8

# NUTRITIONAL SUPPORT – THE LAST PIECE OF THE PUZZLE

In the preceding chapters, I revealed—and you discovered—the value of natural hormone replacement. The benefits were brought to life by the stories of people just like you whose lives were changed and revitalized by fixing their hormone imbalances and not overmedicating each and every symptom.

What we've covered so far is a very good foundation for success. But we're not quite done yet.

The final piece of the puzzle, and the key to facilitating the success of each hormone we optimize, is the nutritional support patients need and should receive through supplementation.

If estrogen works synergistically with testosterone, if thyroid hormone works synergistically with both E and T, then it's the vitamins and minerals I'm going to talk about in this chapter that will help complete your hormone optimization and set you on the path to better health at any age.

The first challenge facing any patient is the huge amount of sometimes accurate, sometimes inaccurate, and sometimes bewildering opinions put forth by doctors and practitioners about nutritional supplements.

Michael Zeligs, M.D., and A. Scott Connelly, M.D., claim in their book *All About DIM,* that "Women and men, athletes and non-athletes alike, are discovering that diindolylmethane (DIM) is the dietary connection to a better metabolism."

"We are all victims of Health Lies. Primary among those lies... is that we need calcium to have strong bones. This is absolutely untrue!" This was elaborated on in *The Calcium Lie* by Robert Thompson, M.D. In 2011, based their analysis of many studies, the prestigious *British Medical Journal* reported that women who took calcium supplements for the prevention of osteoporosis *increased* their risk for atherosclerosis, heart attacks, and strokes.

It seems that every week there is a medical article on Vitamin D. One week it is invaluable. The next it does not benefit the heart and bones. Does Vitamin D need another vitamin to achieve its benefits?

Dr. Kate Rheaume-Bleue, in her book, *Vitamin K2 and the Calcium Paradox,* unravels the mystery by demonstrating that if you have osteoporosis or heart disease, you have vitamin K2 deficiency. Maybe we need both Vitamin D and K2! I will elaborate on that very real possibility later in this chapter.

## IODINE

Let's sort out fact from fiction. The journey into the land of neutraceuticals (a portmanteau of the words "nutrition" and "pharmaceutical") should begin with iodine.

In his book, *Iodine, Why You Need It, Why You Can't live Without It,* David Brownstein, M.D., says, "Iodine is the most misunderstood nutrient."

David Derry, M. D., Ph.D., in his book *Breast Cancer and Iodine*, writes, "Every cell and every fluid in the body contains iodine, so it is surprising to learn few biological textbooks have iodine in their index."

Lynn Farrow, in her book *The Iodine Crisis*, states, "Iodine has become a public health crisis." It's true—this micronutrient is essential to every cell in the body. From the late 1800s to the1960s it was considered the universal medicine, and was used to treat a wide range of diseases including goiter, atherosclerosis, syphilis, uterine fibroids, prostate enlargement, scarlet fever, upper respiratory tract infections (URI), obesity, depression, breast pain, skin conditions, malaria, and a host of others.

Most people associate iodine with the production of thyroid hormone. However, iodine is in fact necessary for the production of *all* hormones. You need iodine if you want your immune system to function at its highest level. Iodine has therapeutic benefits for fibrocystic breast disease, vaginal infections, ovarian disorders and prostate disorders. Iodine is necessary for the normal growth and development of your children. It is the number one cause of preventable mental retardation. Nature has assisted you with this by attaching iodine to the protein secreted in breast milk.

A lack of iodine spells trouble. In 1976, in the journal *Lancet,* the authors reported that iodine deficiency increased the risk of breast, prostate, endometrial, and ovarian cancer.

Amazingly, many humans aren't getting enough of this vital substance. In 1998 the World Health Organization reported that 72% of the world's population is iodine deficient. The Center For Disease Control (CDC) reported in 2000 that iodine consumption had *decreased* 50% since the 1970s. From the seventies until today, breast cancer rates have risen from one in twenty-three to one in seven. Prostate and thyroid diseases have also increased. According to research by Lynne Farrow and explained in her book *The Iodine Crisis*, rates of thyroid cancer have risen 182% between 1975 and 2005.

Iodine deficiency in pregnant women is producing less intelligent children.

## Where Did All the Iodine Go?

What has happened to our iodine in the last half century? In the 1960s, iodine was added to our bread dough. This was a good thing, since one slice of bread gave you your recommended daily allowance. Unfortunately, twenty years later, the National Institute of Health came to believe we were getting too much iodine. This idea was not based on any credible scientific evidence.

In 1980, iodine was removed from bread and was replaced by bromide. This was highly unfortunate, as bromide is toxic. It *purges* iodine from your body. Bromide is found in bread, Gatorade, swimming pools, fire retardant, carpets, furniture, nail polish, and make-up, to name a few items you're in contact with on a daily basis. Bromide toxicity is the underlying cause of the rise in breast cancer. Bromide has been banned in Europe, but not in the United States.

Help! Does anyone know of an antidote for bromide toxicity? After reading this chapter, *you* will know!

In addition, we have depleted iodine from our soils, so our foods have much less of this micronutrient that our bodies demand to function at their highest level. Some areas near the ocean have moderate levels of iodine in the soil; however, the further inland you go, less and less iodine exists in the soil.

For reasons that are difficult to explain, an irrational resistance to iodine has emerged in the medical establishment. In 2002, in his treatise on administering iodine, Dr. Guy Abraham coined the term "iodophobia" to describe this. Specifically, many conventional medical doctors think iodine is damaging to the thyroid. However, this could not be further from the truth. This misguided rhetoric has been disproved by the hundreds of thousands of men and women who have benefitted greatly from this nutrient being added to their hormone optimization program. Iodine *protects* the thyroid!

## Should I Eat More Salt?

I know you're probably thinking, "To get iodine, I'll just eat more iodized salt." Nope. Iodized salt does *not* provide adequate intake for optimal health and disease prevention. Iodine in salt is unstable, and within twenty to forty days after opening the package, table salt will lose up to half of its iodine content through vaporization. Then, of the salt you ingest, only ten percent of the iodine is absorbable. Furthermore, cooking with salt further destroys the available iodine. I highly recommend using sea salt for optimal health rather than one of the commercial products.

## Would Seaweed Fix the Problem?

In Japan, seaweed has long been a traditional source of iodine. But today there are too many pollutants in our seawater to recommend seaweed as a treatment, and anyway, no one foresees Americans suddenly consuming huge amounts of seaweed. And if seaweed is converted into kelp tablets, much of the bioavailability of iodine gets lost.

## The Way Forward

Amidst the controversy and inaccurate reports, there is a clear path. You need iodine, and chances are you're not getting enough. My patients are excited by the fact that not only does testosterone optimization reduce the risk of breast cancer, but iodine supplementation also reduces the risk.

## But how much iodine do we need?

The U.S. Food and Drug Administration (FDA) recommends a daily value (DV) of 150 micrograms (mcg) of iodine for an adult. A microgram is 1/1,000 of a milligram. This level was established during World War Two as the minimum needed to prevent goiter in our soldiers. This amount is inadequate to provide support for thyroid, breasts, prostate, and the immune system. Unfortunately, this inaccurate claim is still being taught in medical schools. In fact, it's exactly what I was taught nearly forty years ago.

It takes a minimum of three milligrams (mg) per day to saturate the thyroid. The thyroid uptakes iodine before *any other tissue gets it*. I hope you can see how really starved we are for iodine and how the government is not truly protecting our health by underestimating our iodine requirements.

In contrast, the Japanese are considered one of the world's longest living people, with an extraordinarily lower incidence of breast, endometrial, and ovarian cancers. Japanese males have a lower incidence of prostate cancer than their US counterparts. A major dietary difference that sets Japan apart from other countries is their high iodine intake, with seaweed the most common source. Researchers estimate that the Japanese iodine intake averages from one to three milligrams per day; some sources claim the figure is as high as 45 milligrams per day.

The world's leading researcher on iodine, Dr. Guy Abraham, recommends that the required intake of iodine should be 13 milligrams per day – just for maintenance.

It was reported at the October 2007 Iodine Conference that studies of over four thousand patients recommended starting with 12.5 mg of Iodoral (Lugol's iodine/iodide combination) and gradually titrate up every two to four weeks until 50 mg daily is achieved. (Iodide is the ion state of iodine, occurring when iodine bonds with another element, such as potassium.) Different tissues prefer iodine versus iodide. The combination is most effective. Selenium, zinc, and Vitamins B2 and B3 are co-factors that assist iodine in doing its job and improving thyroid function. BioTE Medical has a proprietary iodine/iodide formulation that already includes selenium and zinc.

Starting low and adding slow is the best way to initiate iodine into your comprehensive wellness plan. The bromide toxins in your body will soon be flushed out. Occasionally, people feel flu-like symptoms when this occurs. You can avoid this by using a salt loading protocol. Take ½ teaspoon of sea salt in eight ounces of water daily. Increase water intake to flush the bromide from your kidneys. You can also stop your iodine supplement on the weekend and allow your body to catch up on getting rid of bromide toxins. This is called the "pulse dosing strategy".

## Are There Any Side Effects From Iodine?

As with any supplement there can be side effects. The most common is the bromide toxicity, as this harmful toxin is purged from your body. You may feel sluggish or have difficulty concentrating ("brain fog"). The salt loading protocol described above will help significantly in preventing this. Taking weekends off will also be of benefit.

If you are receiving too much iodine, you may develop a rash or headache. To treat this, simply go to the "pulse dosing strategy" and reduce your iodine intake at least by one-half.

## Iodine Testimonial From My Patients

Connie is a forty-five-year-old female who after six months of using iodine according to the protocol above noticed her nails were stronger, her seasonal allergies were improved, and the pain from her fibrocystic disease was gone!

Dan is a fifty-year-old male who after three months of iodine therapy was able to sleep through the night. He no longer needed to get up and urinate twice in the night. His more restful nights improved his energy level and his productivity. As an additional benefit he noticed his ejaculations were stronger and more prolonged, a secondary benefit he had not expected.

Gina is a thirty-five-year-old female who suffered heavy menstrual periods, breast tenderness, and extreme fatigue. One of her doctors had treated her with synthetic thyroid only, and she felt no benefit. I began treatment with Nature-Throid and iodine supplementation with zinc and selenium. She initially felt the bromide detoxification occurring and had forgotten the salt-loading protocol. After adding this simple step into her daily regimen she felt amazing. Her energy was better. Her menstrual periods began lightening. Her breast tenderness decreased significantly.

## DIINDOLYLMETHANE (DIM)

DIM is a phytonutrient, meaning it is a nutrient that comes from plants, specifically cruciferous vegetables like cabbage, broccoli, Brussels sprouts, kale, and cauliflower. It has numerous health benefits for both men and women, and is one of the most important nutrients your body needs to help metabolize your testosterone and estrogen to beneficial byproducts that promote good health. Unfortunately, to obtain therapeutic levels of DIM from food alone you would have to consume large quantities of uncooked vegetables—up to two pounds per day.

For more than twenty years, diindolylmethane has been shown to prevent certain cancers including breast, uterine, and prostate cancer. How does DIM prevent cancer?

Here's how. After estrogen completes its messenger function in your body and the cells, the estrogen begins its prescribed duties, but first has to be metabolized. The metabolites of estrogen are 2-hydroxy estrone, 4-hydroxy estrone, and 16-hydroxy estrone.

The 2-hydroxy estrone is the good metabolite and the one that reduces your chances for cancer. This was first discovered in 1996 by Dr. H. Leon Bradlow.

The 4-hydroxy estrone is the bad metabolite and increases your risk for breast and uterine cancer. This bad estrogen metabolite actually damages the DNA of many of your cells, thus promoting cancer. People who are obese have an increased production of the 4-hydroxy estrone. Many environmental toxins we ingest also increase this bad metabolite.

The 16-hydroxy estrone is intermediate and not effective as an antioxidant or a cancer preventer.

As you may remember from previous chapters, free testosterone is the active form of testosterone in men and women. It has many positive benefits including improving sex drive, mood enhancement, improved sleep, higher energy, and weight loss. DIM enhances estradiol's metabolism to 2-hydroxy estrone.

This estrogen metabolite has the advantage of binding to the protein called sex hormone binding globulin. This process allows testosterone to be released from this protein, and thus your free testosterone is increased. 2-hydroxy estrone also helps fat cells release stored fat.

In men, certain conditions including obesity and excessive alcohol intake increase estradiol. Excessive estradiol increases sex hormone binding globulin. Unfortunately, this leads to increased abdominal obesity, erectile dysfunction, and depressed mood. The good news is that DIM can help metabolize this excess estrogen and help maintain optimal hormone balance.

### Is DIM an Alternative to Hormone Replacement Therapy?
Absolutely not! It is a complementary nutraceutical that makes your hormones safer and reduces their side effects. It is compatible with both estrogen and testosterone therapy. One should think of DIM as completing your hormone optimization.

Is DIM an Aromatase Inhibitor like Femara and Arimidex?

DIM is a natural aromatase inhibitor. It is not as potent as Femara and Arimidex. This makes it a great mild alternative for those men who are only converting a moderate amount of their testosterone to estrogen. By keeping a male's estrogen level optimized you can reduce his risk for atherosclerosis. DIM promotes healthier aging for those males going through andropause who are mild to moderate aromatizers (convert too much of their testosterone to estrogen).

### OK, I'm Ready to Start
Women need 100-200 milligrams of DIM per day. Men need 200-400 milligrams per day. It must be microencapsulated DIM. If it is any other preparation, it will not be absorbed.

Do not be confused by similar products like indole-3-carbinol (I3C). It is often sold next to DIM but is poorly absorbed and has to be converted to DIM in your body. The only patented microencapsulated DIM is made by BIO Response.

**Are There Any Side Effects From DIM?**

There are no reported side effects—another good reason to complete your hormone optimization with DIM.

**Are There Additional Benefits in Patients On Subcutaneous Hormone Pellet Therapy?**

Yes! DIM increases free testosterone in men and women. As a result, it has the potential to make your pellet therapy last longer. This means you will require fewer pellet insertions, realizing a long-term cost savings without sacrificing any benefits.

## VITAMIN D3 AND VITAMIN K2

The next important vitamin supplement is Vitamin D3 (the "sunshine vitamin"). There is a worldwide crisis of D3 deficiency that affects one billion people. Low levels of Vitamin D3 (levels under 60) have been implicated in many different types of cancer including colon, breast, prostate, colorectal, lung, ovarian, esophageal, kidney, and bladder cancer. In the July 2008 issue of the *American Journal of Clinical Nutrition*, the Fred Hutchinson Cancer Research Center in Seattle reported a high incidence of Vitamin D deficiency among female breast cancer survivors. In the *Archives of Internal Medicine* in 2008, low Vitamin D3 was found to be a predictor of all-cause-mortality. Would you want to have low Vitamin D3 and have an increased risk of dying? Of course not, and I will help you avoid that problem.

Vitamin D3 plays a role in moderating or preventing autoimmune conditions such as multiple sclerosis, Type I diabetes, and rheumatoid arthritis.

It's necessary for optimal functioning of your heart. In the Framingham Heart Study, people with Vitamin D3 levels below 15 ng/ml were twice as likely to experience a heart attack, stroke, or other cardiovascular event. Other studies show D levels under 60 hold 160% increased risk of coronary artery disease. Have you ever wondered why there are more heart attacks around the winter holidays? The seasonal lack of sun exposure has been implicated as a probable cause.

Currently, the US recommended daily allowance (RDA) for Vitamin D is 400 IU for the majority of the population to prevent rickets (eradicated in the US, but the federal government has not adjusted the RDA). The Institute of Medicine, the health care arm of the National Academy of Science, only recognizes Vitamin D3 deficiency if blood levels are below 12 ng./ml. or "inadequate" levels if < 20 ng./ml. They are remiss in not recommending the higher levels > 60ng. /ml. required for cancer prevention, heart protection, and reducing mortality.

**How Do Vitamins D3 and K2 Work Together?**
Vitamin D3 has many positive benefits that help protect your bones and heart. Vitamin D3 is vital in producing osteocalcin in your bones. Osteocalcin is a protein secreted in bones that assists with remodeling your bones by both reabsorbing older bone and laying down new healthy bone.

Vitamin D3 also enhances muscle strength and improves balance. People with low levels of Vitamin D3 can have muscle weakness and muscle pain. In fact, if you have an injury to your muscle, Vitamin D3 reduces the time for healing.

It is a vital nutrient and works synergistically with testosterone, estrogen, and thyroid hormone to reduce osteoporosis and fractures. It has a vital role in your heart by reducing plaque formation in the heart's blood vessels. This allows better oxygenation of the heart muscle. It also helps prevent hypertension and thereby protecting the heart in this manner also.

Vitamin D3 cannot do it all alone. It needs help from Vitamin K2, also known as menaquinone. An important fat-soluble vitamin that plays critical roles in protecting your heart, bones, brain, Vitamin K2 also aids in cancer protection.

It actually activates the osteocalcin made by the osteoblast in the bone. Thus Vitamin D3 and Vitamin K2 are partner co-factors in protecting your bones. The biological role of Vitamin K2 is to help move calcium into the proper areas in your body, such as your bones and teeth.

More than half of Americans develop osteoporosis after age fifty. Millions of women and men suffer hip fractures because of osteoporosis. Yes, I said men. They actually account for twenty percent of patients with this disorder of the bones. Research shows that you are five times more likely to have a hip fracture if you are low on Vitamin K2. For those patients who require a total knee replacement or total hip replacement, if you have osteoporosis you have a forty percent chance of needing a repeat surgery. Maintaining strong healthy bones reduces the chances for having a repeat surgery significantly.

If you take a calcium supplement, it's important to maintain the proper balance between calcium, Vitamin K2, and Vitamin D3. Calcium alone does little to nothing to prevent osteoporosis. Adding vitamin D3 is helpful, but the most significant improvements are seen by adding the missing link: Vitamin K2.

Vitamin K2 helps remove calcium from areas where it shouldn't be, such as in your arteries and soft tissues. As was reported in the journal *Atherosclerosis* in 2009, it's the most important nutritional supplement in preventing and even reducing those life-robbing plaques in your heart. This means just what it sounds like: you can reverse heart disease by maintaining adequate blood levels on Vitamin K2. If you take oral Vitamin D, you also need to take Vitamin K2. Vitamin K2 deficiency is actually what produces the symptoms of Vitamin D toxicity, which includes inappropriate calcification that can lead to hardening of your arteries.

To achieve the healthy blood levels of Vitamin D3, adults need a *minimum* of 5,000 IU of D3 daily and up to 10,000 IU daily. Interestingly, every day I see patients who are taking 1,000 units of Vitamin D3 and they believe they are taking a "high dose."

Vitamin K2 dosing has not been well established according to the literature; however, what we do know is that 120 micrograms (mcg) per day is the minimum. Some research shows it takes up to 500 mcg to achieve the needed levels to shuttle calcium into the bones and teeth, where it belongs.

Are There Any Side Effects From D3?

At the recommended doses, side effects from Vitamin D3 are rare. At higher doses patients have reported increased thirst, diarrhea, and muscle aches. If you take Vitamin D3 *without* Vitamin K2, you have an increased risk of hypercalcemia (too much calcium in your blood stream), leading to kidney stones.

## A PERSONAL NOTE

My father was fifty-five years old when he developed aortic stenosis, a narrowing of the large artery exiting the heart. His conventional medical doctors tried medications, but the narrowing progressed. He became short of breath. They recommended surgery to replace the valve. The life expectancy of these surgically replaced valves is often ten years. The second surgery is often fatal. In his sixties he again became short of breath. After undergoing the second surgery, he passed away.

It was about four years later that forward-thinking cardiologists began actively using Vitamin K2 to reverse the narrowing of the aorta by significant amounts without surgery. I wish my father had been treated by one of these cardiologists.

CHAPTER 9

# TO AGE HEALTHIER, FIND THE RIGHT PRACTITIONER

If you're reading this chapter, you've come a long way. I know you feel terrible that the soldiers in your medicine cabinet, the drugs designed to treat ailments that were often preventable, have held you hostage, not allowing you to enjoy the seasons of your life in the most happy and productive way possible.

Healthcare is changing. You are now a large impetus to the paradigm shift. The opportunities to partner with your physician are expanding.

Millions of people just like you are able to rid themselves of medications they do not need. Television ads are no longer captivating you. You view with disdain the magazine ads for the latest pills to cure what does *not* ail you.

In the previous chapters you've experienced a wondrous journey into healthy aging and natural hormone replacement. You've also read about many of my patients whose lives have changed by the therapy I offered them. My greatest reward has been in gifting this knowledge to other healthcare providers and watching them change both their own lives and those of their patients.

Of the hundreds of inspiring journeys and testimonials I've witnessed, I'd like to share six of them with you. These testimonials have been written not by me, but by the doctors and patients themselves. Here are their stories.

## MARCY HENSON, CNFP, PROSPER, TEXAS

In 2009, I spent a great deal of time researching bio-identical hormone replacement. I started offering pellet therapy for my patients and experienced very positive results. In 2011, I had the opportunity to start my own practice. This was a risky venture because I did not have a personal base of patients to sustain a new practice. We opened as a small, single provider office in a small town in North Texas with about a hundred loyal patients receiving pellet therapy, and quickly exceeded our expectations of growth.

Today we have patients from many towns in Texas over three hundred miles away (Texas is a big state!) and from eight neighboring states. Many loyal patients routinely drive more than an hour each way to receive care in our office. We have outgrown our office and are maxed to capacity with six-week waiting lists for new patients. To accommodate our growth we're building a new office with an additional three thousand square feet. We're looking forward to our upcoming expansion, adding more services and providers, and increasing the capacity to care for patients.

We have built our medical practice in a very unconventional way. We don't advertise. Why? Because pellet therapy patients are walking advertisements. All of our patients come from direct referrals and word of mouth. Most of our patients present for a consult for pellet therapy, but once they learn that we are a full service family practice, they decide to transfer all of their medical care.

The greatest part of this journey has not been watching the rapid explosion of growth within our practice; it has been watching peoples' lives change forever. We have patients who were in the process of filing for divorce and, after treatment, sent us flowers as a thank-you for saving their marriage. We have a patient who has a brain tumor, and his neuro-oncologist sent him to us to get testosterone pellets while he was receiving chemotherapy. This patient has received chemotherapy every other week for three years without ever having his blood counts drop or missing work for fatigue. His neurosurgeon and oncologist are thrilled with his progress, endurance, and strength.

We are honored to be part of his journey, as well as all of our patients' life journeys. We take pride in bringing joy back into peoples' lives and helping them feel their best, so they can live their life to the fullest.

## PATIENT & PHYSICIAN TESTIMONIALS

**Diane K.**

After suffering from menopausal symptoms for a number of years, unfortunately with increasing severity, I decided to seek hormone replacement therapy as an option for relief. I researched and considered traditional methods, but was concerned about side effects of the more common remedies. I heard from a coworker about the BioTE method of optimizing all my hormones, and made an appointment with Marcy to discuss my options. Marcy told me about the BioTE alternative and explained the treatment method and benefits.

I made the decision to begin BioTE immediately. Within six weeks after my initial treatment I started feeling more like I did when I was forty than in my early fifties. I was more energetic, my ill temper and moodiness dissipated, my libido was vastly improved, and my overall health was noticeably better.

It has been over three years now since I began BioTE, and I fully credit it and Marcy for making my life so much more enjoyable. My co-workers, husband, and children all comment about how much more like "myself" I have been since I started the BioTE treatments. I have maintained a twenty-five-pound weight loss, continue to have an energy level that I never dreamed I would have at fifty-six, and have absolutely none of the miserable menopause symptoms I had before starting BioTE. I have and will continue to recommend this treatment to anyone. It really was a life-changing experience for me.

**Lisa Jukes, *M. D., Gynecologist, Austin, Texas***
If anyone had told me ten years ago that I would be using implantable hormones in my patients, I would not have believed them. I was trained conservatively at the University of Texas Southwestern Medical School for both medical school and ob/gyn residency. After graduating in 2000, I moved to Austin. I transitioned from a group into a solo practice in 2004, and later that year stopped obstetrics so that I could focus on comprehensive gynecologic care and minimally invasive surgery.

Over the years, my patients were transitioned (typically from Prempro) to transdermal estrogens creams and patches, bio-identical progesterone, and occasionally Estratest, if needing help with their libido.

While my office had earned a reputation of up-to-date, patient-oriented, detailed care by myself and mid-level providers, I noticed that patients were sometimes going elsewhere to see "hormone experts." Unfortunately, patients were also not being managed well, and in some situations had inadequately opposed estrogen with transdermal progesterones or no progesterone at all. After two such patients developed uterine cancer, I queried them as to why they put their health in my hands for gynecologic care but not hormonal management. The answer was that they still did not feel good on the conventional hormonal approach we had tried, and in particular they had no sex drive.

It was time for me to look outside my comfort zone and look into safe ways to address their sense of wellness and help them enjoy their menopausal lives. When I was approached by the BioTE Medical liaison, the timing was right, the company had years of experience, and most importantly, a safe, responsible approach to the application of hormone optimization.

My patients have benefitted from this addition, and I know that I am a better provider with a more comprehensive knowledge of hormones. Furthermore, it has been a positive experience to collaborate with Dr. Gary Donovitz and his team, and have the opportunity to provide feedback on ways to administer natural hormones safely and effectively.

One of my patients, a dental professional, developed breast cancer in her mid-forties. She was diagnosed under my care with breast cancer and then, secondary to other gynecologic concerns, she required a complete hysterectomy. Surgical menopause following chemotherapy was especially challenging for her, with mental fogginess, low energy, night sweats, interrupted sleep, mood interruptions, and of course, low sexual desire. With the consent of her oncologist, she has been using testosterone pellets for nearly two years. I saw her this past week for her fourth round of pellets, and she and I both agree that she looks—and, more importantly, *feels*—better than she has in years, even prior to the cancer. How can we not feel good about offering testosterone to these breast cancer survivors who have the rest of their lives to truly "live"?

Another patient transitioned to my office in Austin from the Dallas area. She was on pellets and was having postmenopausal bleeding. For at least two years she had been receiving excessive estrogen, and then an oral combination non-bio-identical hormone therapy for years prior to the pellets. Hormone therapy misuse led to her developing a cancer in her uterus. A gynecologic oncologist and myself performed her complete da Vinci robotic hysterectomy and removed the pelvic lymph nodes. She is doing well and continues now with testosterone pellets only. She is in her early sixties and feels great. She can only go three months between pellets; otherwise she has night sweats, fatigue and difficulty sleeping. She said again that she does not know what she would do without the testosterone pellets.

There are so many positive patient stories that I can reflect upon—indeed, so much more than with conventional, FDA-approved regimens (bio-identical or not). I used to really believe that low sex drive in women was related to personal issues including stress, over-commitment, relationships, or depression. Like the American College of Obstetrics and Gynecology, I had recommended counseling as a viable treatment option. I now know that while decreased libido is oftentimes multifactorial, low testosterone is a very real and large contributor to the low sex drive that is rampant in society.

It is alarming to see the number of people aged thirty and over with undetectable testosterone levels. As I was once in that category, I cannot imagine going without testosterone pellets myself. It is exciting to offer estrogen and testosterone pellets to patients from a manufacturer that receives FDA oversight and under the guidance of BioTE, a company that is consistently striving to improve outcomes and minimize risks by refining protocols and improving products. It has truly been rewarding to have BioTE as a part of my practice.

**G. DeAn Strobel, *M.D., Fellow, American College of Obstetrics and Gynecology, Sherman, Texas***
As a board-certified ob/gyn, I have been treating postmenopausal and perimenopausal patients since 1999. In 2006, I began delving into the art of bio-identical hormone replacement. I found hormone replacement therapy to be somewhat complicated and frustrating. Many women would have improvement in some of their symptoms (like the vasomotor symptoms) yet have little to no improvement in symptoms of sexual dysfunction and cognition. Others would have significant side effects from hormone therapy such as headaches, severe breast tenderness, or mood swings, and would not want to continue therapy. The fact that there were no known standards or normal ranges made hormone replacement even more difficult.

After having some personal struggles with hormonal deficiencies and less-than-stellar results using bio-identical hormone creams, I decided to find out more about bio-identical hormone pellets. It was at this point that I was introduced to BioTE. I later met Dr. Gary Donovitz and began to learn more about the differences that BioTE pellet therapy offers. While I was excited about the opportunity to try something that would benefit my patients in many ways, I had a healthy amount of skepticism as well.

Within a few short weeks, I realized that the BioTE bio-identical pellet therapy was helping my patients in ways that no other therapy had. I began getting patient calls telling me that they felt better than they had in years. Others would call telling me that BioTE had saved their marriage. Never before in my practice had I received such dramatic phone calls!

Many patients are already aware that testosterone therapy improves sexual function, but many are unaware of the other benefits. I think some of the happiest patients are the patients who, prior to coming to my office, have felt that their memory was slowly declining. After achieving hormonal balance, most of these patients are gratified to report that their memory and cognition are back to normal.

Other patients suffer from severe joint or muscle pain. One particular male patient was scheduled for a knee replacement. He had many symptoms suggestive of low testosterone but had never been tested. He was found to have a testosterone level of about 180 (very low for a male) and was treated with BioTE hormone pellet therapy. Within a few short weeks, he cancelled his knee surgery. Today he reports that he is able to do things he hasn't done in many years and is almost pain-free. Of course, I do not advocate such dramatic results in most severely arthritic patients, but I have seen significant improvement in pain from arthritis as well as pain from fibromyalgia in several of my patients.

Another frustrating symptom that I have seen over the years in patients of all ages is that of fatigue. Fatigue is such a common complaint that clinicians often overlook it. Most clinicians will check blood counts and thyroid labs. If those values are normal, usually the patient is told that his or her symptoms are likely due to stress or depression. In contrast—once other underlying causes are carefully ruled out—when the patient is brought to hormonal balance, fatigue is almost assuredly resolved.

As a gynecologist, I have found vulvar lichen sclerosis to be a difficult disease to treat. Several patients over the years have presented with such discomfort that they are limited to wearing loose cotton panties with skirts. Many are too uncomfortable to even wear the loosest pants. I have found most of the patients to return to normal within a few months. I usually encourage at least six to nine months of BioTE hormone therapy for these patients and have had an excellent response. I have not had this type of response with any of the topical steroid creams in the past (estrogen, testosterone, or steroid).

Finally equipped with something that actually works to help relieve the symptoms of hormonal imbalances, I feel very happy to offer my patients BioTE hormone therapy. I would say that up to ninety percent of my patients have positive results and are pleased with how they feel. Never before have I had such wonderful results from a hormone therapy.

**Steven Komadina, *M.D., Board Certified Obstetrician-Gynecologist, Albuquerque, New Mexico***
For years I watched while patients traveled hundreds of miles to get their pellets for hormone replacement in the menopausal period of life. I frankly thought they were a little crazy, but they tried to convince me that it was like night and day versus what I had done with creams, gels, troches, pills, and patches.

Many such patients were longtime friends, and I finally decided I needed to know more. I flew to Dallas. After meeting with Dr. Gary Donovitz I decided the science was beyond reproach and the results were impossible to argue with. I started down the path of true bio-identical replacement with pellets delivered in a customized dose in the right way and to the right person.

Over a thousand patients later, the results speak for themselves. Here is a perfect example:

Mary Ann is a sixty-year-old menopausal mother of three, married to a physician. She never planned on hormone replacement, as she preferred to let nature take its course. At her husband's insistence she attended an evening lecture on the value of hormone balance. She then agreed to pellet hormone replacement with estrogen and testosterone pellets and oral progesterone to balance the estrogen effect on the uterus.

That decision changed her life. Her excitement was incredible as the replacement took effect. Energy up, sleep perfect, joint pain gone, night sweats gone, hot flashes gone, mental clarity sharp, mood even—and then there was libido. This wonderful couple had been married for forty years and had wonderful children who had all been planned because Mary Ann never had any libido. Intercourse was what you did to get pregnant. This aspect of their marriage never was fulfilled, but their devotion to each other solidified their love without a sexual component.

Within two weeks of pellet therapy all that changed! As she described it.... "It wasn't a lust, but true love. For the first time in forty years I could not wait to be held, cuddled and then consummate that experience with wonderful physical contact. I had never experienced anything like this in my life."

As a physician, this opportunity to truly change the quality of life is precious, and adding pellet therapy to my bag of medical therapies has been a tremendous experience for me as well as my patients.

**Denise Pollard, *APRN-C, Omaha, Nebraska***
I am a board certified Women's Health Nurse Practitioner and began practicing OB/GYN in 2007. During that time, I saw women every day that were mismanaged by their other providers and their symptoms were never truly addressed. Most of the time these women were placed on antidepressants, sleeping pills, and anti-anxiety medication that only masked their symptoms. It was in 2009 that I decided that I needed to step up to help these women and fully address the underlying issues that so many other providers overlooked. I trained under Dr. Gary Donovitz and began treating women with bio-identical hormone pellet therapy. It has been a blessing to my patient's health and their quality of life to have this type of therapy available to them.

Nearly three years ago, I met a lovely woman named Koanne. She traveled 2-1/2 hours to see me from Grand Island, NE. Initially, she complained of extreme fatigue and was frustrated that no one was addressing this for her. After digging a little deeper into her medical history, I discovered this 52-year-old female suffered from severe daily migraine headaches. She was having to spend most of her day lying in bed due to the severity of her headaches. It seemed that they were taking over her life and this is how she would live. I reviewed all of her lab levels and balanced her thyroid, vitamins, and hormones. Within weeks she was noticing improvements. She was feeling more energetic, but even more importantly, she had not had a migraine since her first treatment with me. I have seen her for nearly three years and she remains migraine-free. She is now able to enjoy her life to the fullest by traveling with her husband and riding his motorcycle with him. She has even been caught skydiving and going to Sturgis! Koanne is truly experiencing a wonderful quality of life due to Bio TE and pellet therapy and I am so happy I was involved in helping her.

### Terri Suresh, *RN, MSN, ACNP, Southlake, Texas*

In 2008 I found myself in a dilemma. I had been working in the hospital as an emergency and internal medicine practitioner, taking care of emergent and non-emergent hospitalized patients. I was noticing a trend that was not sitting well with me: Too many patients seemed to be on the same drugs, for the same reasons, with the same doses in most cases, and almost always without relief of symptoms. I had become a medical practitioner to diagnose, prevent, and heal disease, and I was becoming more and more dissatisfied with my job. It seemed that we practitioners were spending most of our time managing prescriptions and symptoms, and no one was looking at the "why."

I wanted to know why.

- Why were ninety percent of my patients exhausted, overweight, and depressed?
- Why were so many patients on medications for type 2

diabetes, heart disease, high cholesterol, and high blood pressure? Weren't these disease processes preventable?

• Why were patients placed on medications and just told to "exercise more" and "eat right"?

• Why were so many people being told their thyroid was "normal" because their labs were "normal" – but they still had all of the symptoms of low thyroid? Every time I would round on a hospitalized patient, or see a patient with these vague complaints in the emergency room and I gave them the same spiel everyone else was, I felt it was wrong.

My intuition told me there had to be a better way to care for patients. I decided at that moment—at two in the morning in the emergency room—that I was going to find some answers. I had heard stories about the miracles of bio-identical hormone replacement therapy (BHRT) in women, so I did some research before attending an anti-aging conference to learn more about this life-altering therapy.

I opened up my first hormone clinic in a small room I rented at a salon, and started the process of educating women on the importance of hormone balance. The problem was the training I was doing on creams only helped in a small percentage of women, namely, menopausal women having hot flashes—and when they did work it was only for a short time. No one was teaching about testosterone therapy in women or addressing the pre-menopausal years—those years from thirty to fifty during which we suffer from depression, irritability, mood swings, brain fog, extreme fatigue, low sex drive, and a host of other symptoms. The progesterone cream I prescribed for the women who had those symptoms just wasn't working. Moreover, every time I went to a bio-identical hormone conference and asked how to read saliva test results and dose according to deficiencies, I was met with confusing answers and basically a... "just try a little more of this or that." This seemed worse than giving prescriptions for antidepressants and sleeping pills! I felt like

I was back to square one, with more of the same guesswork instead of fixing the problem.

About six months after I started my BHRT cream clinic, I had a few patients contact me to see if I was doing pellet therapy yet. I hadn't heard of pellets and I certainly had never heard of giving women testosterone, but based on the feedback from my patients, this was something I thought I'd better figure out quickly! Several of my patients had transferred under the care of Dr. Gary Donovitz, so I decided to meet with him and figure out what all of the hubbub was about.

After meeting with Dr. Donovitz and understanding how important testosterone is in both women and men, and how the pellet therapy is dosed specifically to the patient based on lab values, symptoms, and a host of other factors, all of the unanswered questions became clear. I decided at that moment to become trained and certified in BHRT pellet method and the rest is history.

I started educating my cream and oral BHRT patients about this amazing alternative and every single one who transitioned never wanted to go back. This therapy *worked*! And talk about simple! Only three or four times per year for women and two or three times per year for men; the steady dose of hormones available 24/7 to the body; no roller coaster effect and minimal-to-no side effects.

What an amazing alternative! The stories of life change abound and have not stopped coming. Every week I have a new one to tell and it makes my job so rewarding. What an incredible space to be in, actually healing people—the entire reason I became a medical practitioner in the first place.

Several stories stand out in my head, but one story stands out particularly. A woman in her sixties whose daughter had been coming to us for treatment finally agreed to be seen. Her husband, in his eighties, is a retired gynecologist desperate to get his wife some help. We did the consultation and deemed her a great candidate for the therapy. A few weeks later when she came in for follow-up labs I greeted her in the hallway and asked her how she was doing, at which point she began to cry. My first thought was I didn't get her hormones balanced very well! But when she regained her composure she said simply this: "For twenty-five years, I have not liked my husband. Now I realize it was me and not him. I feel like I have lost all of this time with him." She felt incredible, like her old self from thirty years earlier—increased energy, moods stable, focus and mental clarity returned, joint pain gone, vaginal pain and dryness gone, and a sex drive to boot! She lamented the loss of time with her husband, and having been too wrapped up in her own misery that she did not realize what a gift she had in him.

A few weeks later I went in to see my next patient, and lo and behold, it was her husband, the retired gynecologist. He stated, "Before we get started, I want to tell you that had I known about this therapy when I was a practicing gynecologist, based on the changes I have seen in my wife, I would have placed every woman on it. Thank you for giving me my wife back." He lamented the loss of time as well—time healing his patients, particularly his own wife, and giving them a quality of life once thought unattainable after a certain age.

The stories go on and on. Thousands of my patients, aged twenty to one hundred, have benefited from this life-changing therapy. As a practitioner and patient of the therapy myself, I feel incredibly blessed to have met Dr. Donovitz and to have learned how to heal and give people an opportunity to heal and be fully present in all aspects of their lives, not only from a physical and symptom relief standpoint, but spiritual, emotional and most importantly, relationship healing. Countless patients have and will continue to benefit from this amazing therapy!

The collective journey of so many healthcare practitioners and their patients confirms that healthcare is changing. The new focus is on the health and vitality of our patients. Practitioners are seeing other practitioners happy in their chosen field for the first time in years. The goal of healthy aging has been elusive as physicians, insurance companies, and big pharmaceutical companies have engaged in marketing warfare benefitting no one and decimating the quality of life of too many patients. The benefits are amazing as seen from the testimonials.

Your life should not be held hostage by expensive medications that mask symptoms. It's meant to be full of vitality and the energy of youth. The lesson is to find the right practitioner! Do not let days turn into weeks into months into years. Let the power of healing hormones give you back your life.

CHAPTER 10

# THE HEALING POSSIBILITIES ARE ENDLESS

A pebble hits the glass-like surface of a pond, and the ripples fan out like rings of life farther and farther from where the pebble entered. We've all seen a picture of this and have wondered at its meaning.

The benefits to natural hormone replacement therapy are numerous and life changing. When I cast the pebble with all the ways peoples' lives can be changed and aging made healthier, I see the *rings of life* expanding and getting larger and larger.

So what do they mean?

They are promises of hope to those who could benefit from hormone optimization. Hope for mothers of multiple babies. Hope for breast cancer survivors. Hope for athletes who have sustained traumatic brain injuries (TBI) from concussions. Hope for the veterans who return from war with post-traumatic stress disorder (PTSD).

You know that conventional medicine remains lost in the forest, unable to appreciate or fully accept the benefits of hormone replacement therapy. Knowledge is power; and if the information I have shared with you remains elusive to those mired in the fog of conventional medicine, then they have rendered themselves powerless to care for those in need today, and those described below who will need help in the future.

## MOTHERS OF MULTIPLES

You probably would not think that mothers of multiple babies (MOMs) would be a subset of people interested or in need of hormone replacement therapy. MOM was a term rarely talked about until after the turn of the millennium.

The first "test tube baby" was born in 1978. It was then the opportunity arose for infertile couples to achieve their life's dreams of a baby, and even of multiple babies. Since 1981, hundreds of thousands of babies have been born as a result of this technique. Many of them are twins and triplets.

However, even without infertility treatments, more and more women are giving birth to twins. This phenomenon has sparked much speculation. Reasons given for this increase in twin births include:

- Women getting pregnant at an older age.
- Women using birth control pills for many years, then stopping the pill, and getting pregnant within the first few weeks of fertility.
- Women who already have kids and now shooting for number three (and being blessed with three and four).
- Family history.

The mothers of these special bundles of joy have needs that are clearly not being met. To achieve these in-vitro fertilization pregnancies, injections of medications are used to stimulate eggs in the ovary to grow. Those multiple excited eggs produce excessive amounts of hormones, often exceeding the amounts produced by their somewhat poorly functioning ovary. The process is stressful, costly, and involves a roller coaster ride (literally—ask any female fertility patient!) of hormone changes and emotions.

However, even without the injections, the family is faced with challenges they were not prepared for. MOMs have hormone imbalances that are radical. These lead to problems including insomnia, mood swing, irritability, fatigue, weight gain, and lower sex drives. They are subjected to a balancing act between spouse and kids often with no preparation. The mother of multiples' friends and contemporaries may be having a more protracted change in their hormones allowing time for the body to adjust. Mothers of multiples also face higher rates of postpartum depression.

Mothers of multiples often seek out medical attention, which "band aids" the symptoms by obscuring sensory processes using antidepressants. Why would you want to blunt the special time of bonding and nurturing? Is that necessary? Their sex drives, which are already minimized, become nonexistent. Is that healthy for her strained and often disordered marriage? Of course not! Mothers of multiples often cannot sleep. The exhaustion and sleep deprivation caused by nursing two babies at the same time is hard to comprehend unless seen first hand. Their time demands are incredible. Sleep deprivation can lead to mood swings and poor eating habits. Sleeping pills are not the answer—think of the needs of the new babies.

So what do the *rings of life* have to offer mothers of multiples? The answer is that in a women who has had her hormone levels severely compromised, restoring the balance in those hormones will allow her to have an optimal quality of life, an immune system that remains strong, and the mental stamina to enjoy the gifts that have been bestowed upon her. The mothers of multiples will be happy to know they can still nurse their babies and optimize their hormones.

## PATIENT TESTIMONIAL:
## ANDREA J. OF MANSFIELD, TEXAS

After wishing for a little brother for my two girls, everybody around me told me that I must be ecstatic to have given birth to identical twin boys. I felt blessed, yes, but at the same time I felt guilty all the time, as I was not as happy as I felt I should be. I was always tired and had no energy. Besides attending to the boys, I pretty much got nothing done, even when they slept. On top of that I could not get back to my regular size like I did after the first two pregnancies as soon as the girls had been weaned. I was told this was normal, but I did not want to accept that. A friend told me about pellets and how it changed her life. I had my blood checked and my testosterone level was seven. I still remember the practitioner asking me all these questions about my symptoms and explaining to me that I felt the way I did because of my testosterone number being seven, as this is a *very* low level. I have been on pellets for many years now and can honestly say that this is the best thing I have ever done.

I am back to size six, and I was over two hundred pounds during my pregnancy. I am happily married and raising five kids. I go to the gym every morning at five in the morning, and then make my kids' school lunches before I go to a full-time job. I coach little league and am active in my church. Oh—and I am forty-eight years old!

Without pellets, I would not be where I am today.

## BREAST CANCER

The most common of the female cancers, breast cancer, kills approximately four hundred thousand women in the United States every year. How unfair it is for physicians to be withholding the very medicine that confers protection against this disease! How unfair it is for physicians to withhold the very medicines that can improve the quality of life for so many women and expand their lifespans by decades.

In five continents, natural bio-identical testosterone has been used to treat breast cancer. It has been shown to decrease the incidence of the disease and even shrink breast tumors before they were removed.

It is interesting that women fear estrogen. They have been convinced by the media that estrogen causes breast cancer. By definition, "sensationalism" is the spreading of a shocking story or language at the expense of accuracy, solely in order to provoke public interest or excitement. "At the expense of accuracy" should be the definition of media malpractice. Especially when millions of women hear the message that hormones are risker than what is advertised.

The truth remains that estrogen does not cause breast cancer. Really? Did I just say that! It's true! Even in the Women's Health Initiative, using only estrogen, there was no increase in breast cancers. Wow! Where was that on the 5 o'clock news or in *Time* magazine or *The New York Times*? Millions of women would have benefited from that news. Instead, as reported in *The American Journal of Public Health* in 2013, tens of thousands of women died from *estrogen avoidance*.

I'm sure you'll relate to one of my favorite patients, Angela. She was young when afflicted by breast cancer. The disease caused her tremendous stress. After treatment she became depressed and her energy level was low. She even succumbed to using anti-depressants.

She was treated with Tamoxafen, a drug used to reduce the spread of invasive breast cancer. The drug can cause blood clots in the leg and cancer in the womb. She developed a pain in her feet so severe it made walking difficult. She felt the downward spiral in her life, her marriage, and her role as mother to two children.

Was she doomed to be a woman who could barely walk? Whose very life-force energy was nonexistent?

To compound the tragedy, while this was happening, her doctors warned her against hormone replacement therapy.

Nearly three years later she learned her fate was not sealed. It was contained in the *rings of life*. She regained her life with hormone optimization. She had a life beyond breast cancer. Her future was bright, her energy could be restored, and her foot pain could be resolved. Why was she deprived of hormones for too long? They were a lifeline to a future she did not think she had.

A future that was almost taken from her.

Her quality of life is incredible. Her future remains bright. Is she risking her health? No, she is enhancing her health, which is the future she only dreamed of.

This is the future of health and vitality as seen through the eyes of Angela.

## TRAUMATIC BRAIN INJURY (TBI)

Traumatic brain injury (TBI) is a national health problem that leads to disability, death, and neurologic and hormone dysfunction. According to the CDC in 2014, during the decade from 2001 to 2010 the rates of traumatic brain injury (TBI) emergency room visits, hospitalizations, and deaths in the United States increased from 521 per 100,000 to 823 per 100,000. In 2010, 2.5 million TBIs were reported—and given the fact that it's estimated that one-fourth of persons who sustain a TBI do not seek care, the number should be even higher.

The long-term effects of a TBI-related disability include decreased quality of life and persistent medical, social, and economic issues for both the individual and society as a whole. Approximately 3.2 to 5.3 million people live with long-term symptoms from a traumatic brain injury, including the loss of one or more physical or mental capabilities. This is likely an underestimation of the prevalence of TBI due to the high rates of not seeking treatment and the fact that these numbers do not include military injuries. Colleges and college athletic teams also typically under-report their TBI events.

The annual cost of TBI in the United States, including direct medical and rehabilitation costs and indirect societal economic costs, is estimated to be $60 billion dollars (CDC, 2011).

Traumatic brain injury can be described as any change in brain function or other evidence of brain pathology caused by an external force. The alteration in brain function can be expressed as any period or loss of consciousness, any loss of memory for events immediately before or after an injury, neurologic deficits including weakness, loss of balance, visual changes, muscle learning disability, nerve pain, paralysis, sensory loss, aphasia (loss of the ability to communicate verbally), or an alteration in mental state at the time of the injury including confusion, disorientation, or slowed thinking. Evidence of brain pathology can include visual, radiological, or laboratory confirmation of damage to the brain. The external force can include the head being struck by an object, the head striking an object, the brain undergoing an acceleration or deceleration movement without direct external trauma to the head, a foreign body penetrating the brain, or forces generated from a blast or explosion. TBI can be diagnosed as mild, moderate, or severe.

TBI can lead to short- and long-term changes in memory and reasoning. TBI may also affect sensations such as touch, taste, and smell. Language abilities including communication, expression, and understanding may suffer after injury, and emotions such as depression, anxiety, and personality changes may result. The National Institutes of Health (NIH) reports that damage from TBI may result in Alzheimer's disease, Parkinson's disease, and other neurologic problems that involve brain function in older populations.

There is a relationship between traumatic brain injury and chronic pituitary dysfunction leading to multiple hormone imbalances including testosterone and growth hormone. Traumatic brain injuries, such as the kind caused by blast injuries in a military context, can cause hypopituitarism, which we discussed in Chapter 7. The pituitary gland produces six different hormones that help regulate growth, blood pressure, metabolism, temperature, pain, sex organ function, and some aspects of pregnancy and childbirth. People with hypopituitarism are typically deficient in three or more hormones.

According to a 2005 study in the *European Journal of Endocrinology*, post-injury hypopituitarism affects approximately forty percent of people who suffer a traumatic brain injury.

As reported in *Frontiers of Neurology* in 2012, by six months post-TBI, the pituitary deficits and hormone deficiencies present are considered to be relatively permanent.

Several factors may contribute to the hormonal suppression that is typical of the post-TBI patient's experience. Injury to the blood vessels that supply sensitive areas of the brain and compression from swelling are common initiating factors. Symptoms similar to those suffering with PTSD include fatigue, anxiety, depression, irritability, sexual dysfunction, cognitive deficits, and decreased quality of life. Long-term problems include muscle weakness, osteoporosis, decreased energy and motivation, reduced lean body mass, and premature mortality secondary to cardiovascular disease (*Lancet*, 2001). A study of men who had endured severe TBI by Wagner et al. in 2012 found that in the early phase, 100% of participants experienced severe hormone deficits. This persisted in 36% of the victims. Those who had persistent deficiencies in hormone levels were found to have worse functional and cognitive outcomes both six months and twelve months post-injury.

As discussed previously, the benefits of testosterone replacement have been well researched and documented in areas such as self-esteem, libido, decreased irritability and fatigue, and increased muscle strength and bone mineral density. The potential benefits of testosterone therapy in post-TBI patients involve optimization of the physical and psychological recovery.

The benefits are seen in a patient of mine named Alan. He is a fifty-four-year-old man with a history of TBI that began at age twenty-two. For three years, Alan complained of weakness, weight loss, fatigue, lethargy, irritability, decreased appetite, and sexual dysfunction. Blood test revealed his pituitary hormones were low. He was treated with testosterone, thyroid hormone, and hydrocortisone as replacement therapy and showed miraculous improvement in his symptoms.

Failure to identify hormone deficiencies in TBI patients has extremely detrimental consequences. Patients who are out of hormone balance and remain untreated suffer poor quality of life, abnormal body composition, and abnormal blood parameters of healthy metabolism. The importance of this imbalance in the overall health of the individual was elaborated in 2007 in the *Journal of Clinical Endocrinology*. Hormonal replacement and balance may be able to reduce the morbidity and mortality associated with TBI, and should be investigated as an integral piece of the patient's rehabilitation.

## POST-TRAUMATIC STRESS DISORDER (PTSD)

PTSD was first brought to the attention of the medical community by war veterans. It was historically referred to as "shell shock" and "battle fatigue syndrome." The consequences of this disorder affect thousands of veterans and their families.

For a person with PTSD, the symptoms of irritability, insomnia, sexual dysfunction, anxiety, and detachment are persistent. These can become so strong that they keep the person from living a normal life. Conventional medicine continues to battle the disorder using what's known euphemistically as the *bottles of soldiers* in the medicine cabinet—antidepressants, sleeping pills, and memory aids that resemble amphetamines. Ask the war veterans themselves if the quality of their lives is better? If they feel like they have normal lives? If their home life and careers have been enhanced by pills, pills and more pills? The resounding answer is *no*!

Veterans returning from Afghanistan or Iraq have often experienced blast concussions in combat, and many exhibit symptoms indicative of post-traumatic stress disorder.

According to preliminary new research presented at the Experimental Biology 2013 meeting in Boston, there may be a hormonal explanation for the PTSD symptoms.

Nearly half of veterans with blast injuries in the new study had low levels of pituitary hormones, which have been associated with symptoms similar to PTSD, but are simpler to treat.

In the Dutch study reported in the journal Psychoendocrinology in 2014, they looked at 918 males before and after deployment to Afghanistan. Deployment increases testosterone, which is a great thing in maintaining readiness for the travails of combat. In the males with low testosterone pre-deployment, they found a higher incidence of PTSD at one and six months after return. This establishment of who might and more probably would be vulnerable to PTSD may be treatable.

In the journal *Biological Psychiatry* in 2012, researchers found women are twice as likely to develop PTSD as men. It was determined that low estrogen levels in women contributed to the increased incidence. Remember PTSD is not just a product of war, but victims of traumatic crimes and events are also afflicted.

It appears, therefore, that optimizing men's testosterone and maintaining women's estrogen levels in an optimal range may be the novel approach needed to improve symptoms of PTSD and achieve the renewed quality of life for which these patients are striving.

# CHAPTER 11

# HEALTHY AGING MADE SIMPLE

## THE RECIPE FOR HEALTHY AGING

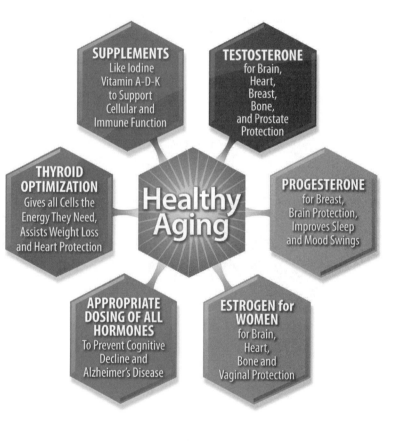

## About Dr. Donovitz

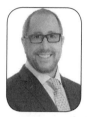 Dr. Donovitz is the C.E.O. and founder of BioTE Medical, LLC. He has been a leading innovator in bio-identical hormone replacement for 20 years. He is a champion of changing healthcare through an individualized, comprehensive method of hormone optimization. He is an expert and international lecturer in subcutaneous hormone pellet therapy, having performed more than 50,000 pellet insertions and having successfully taught the technique to nearly 1,000 practitioners nationwide.

Additionally, Dr. Donovitz has been a pioneer in robotic surgery and has trained physicians across the country on how to perform operations using this procedure.

He received the Isadore Dyer award for best teaching resident while studying at Tulane University in New Orleans, Louisiana. He is a fellow in the American College of Obstetrics and Gynecology, a fellow in the Royal Society of Medicine, and the current medical director for the Institute for Hormonal Balance.

Dr. Donovitz and BioTE Medical are committed to changing healthcare and helping people feel better regardless of age. Its central tenet is that hormone balance offers a genuine opportunity for people to have more successful careers, better relationships, and more productivity through the seasons of their lives.